The Complete Keto Diet Desserts Recipes

50 Fast, Simple, and Tasty Recipes to Stay Fit for Women Over 50

Rose Pope

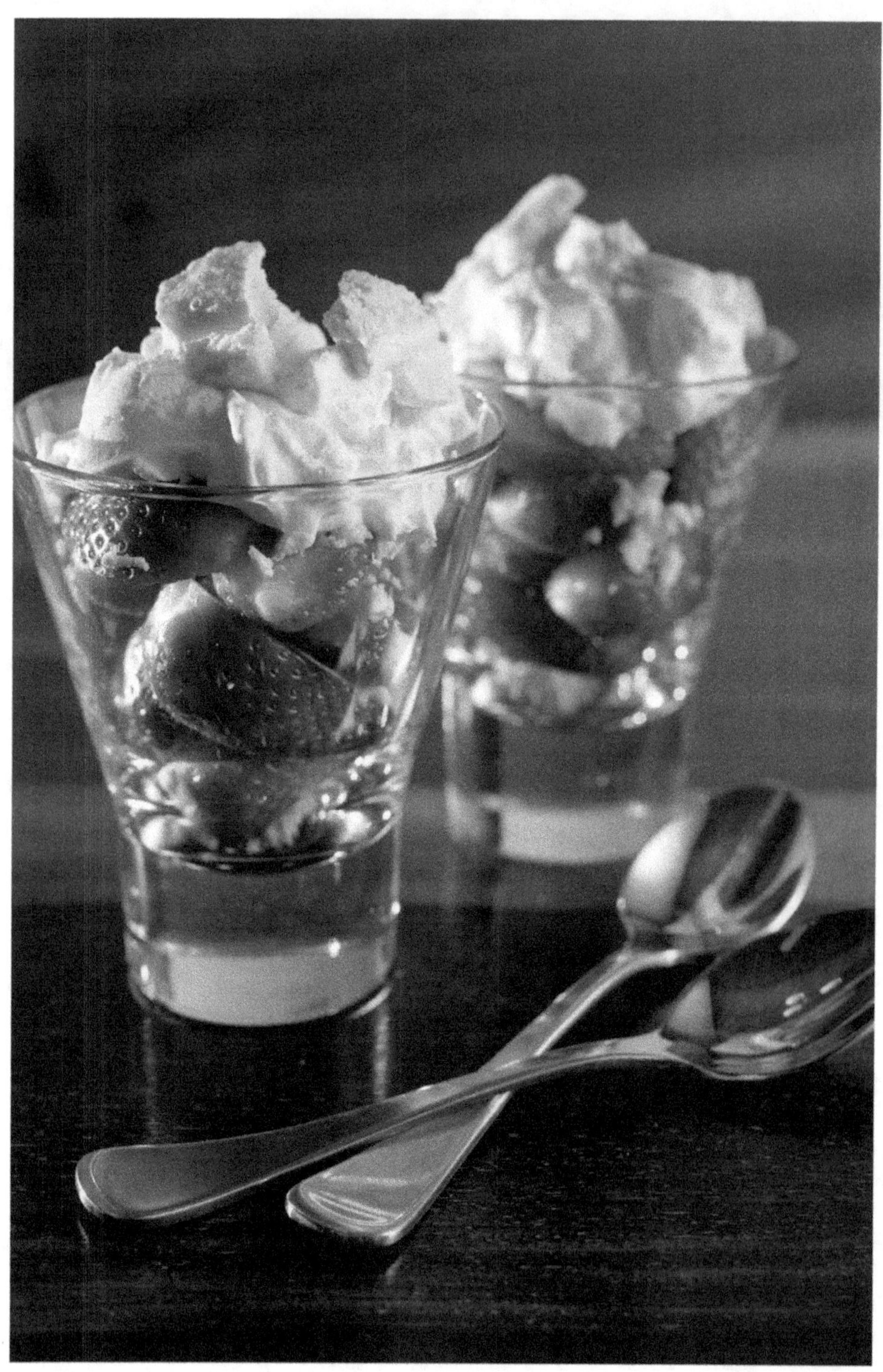

Table of Contents

50 Essential Desserts Recipes

1 Sugar-Free Keto Blueberry Muffins With Almond Flour

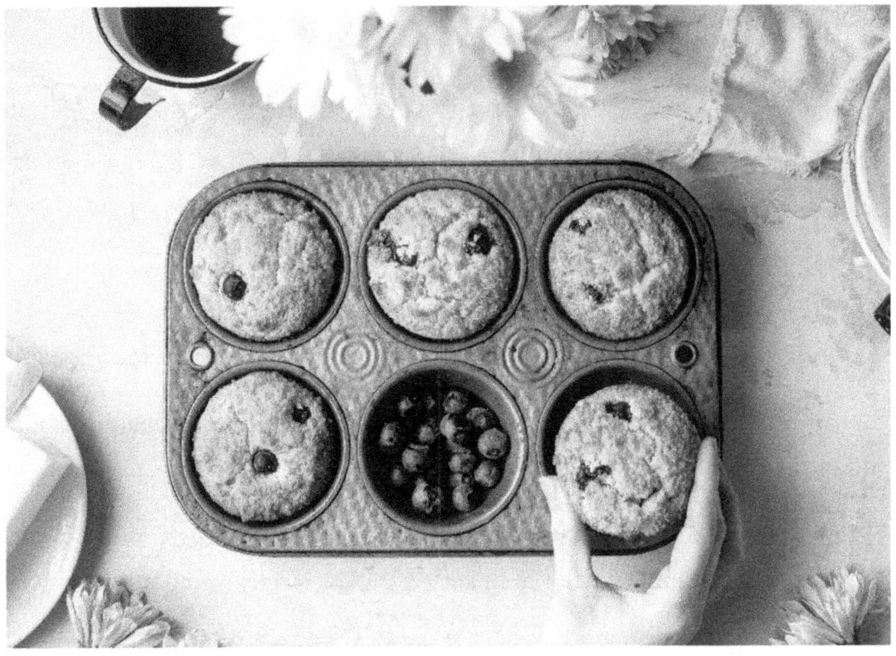

Servings: 12 | **Time**: 45 mins | **Difficulty**: Easy

Nutrients per serving: Calories: 247 kcal | Fat: 21.8g | Carbohydrates: 9.3g | Protein: 7.3g | Fiber: 3.9g

Ingredients

1 Tbsp of Baking powder

1 tsp of Sea salt

1/2 Cup Unsweetened Applesauce

2 tsp Vanilla extract

2/3 Cup Fresh blueberries

3 Cups Almond flour

1 tsp Baking soda

3 Large Eggs, at room temperature

3/4 cup of Monkfruit (or granulated sweetener of choice)

4 Tbsp Coconut flour, packed

7 Tbsp Coconut oil, melted

Method

1. Preheat the oven to 350 F and use an oil spray to spray a muffin pan.

2. Mix the coconut flour, almond flour, baking powder, baking soda, and salt in a medium dish. Just put aside.

3. In a wide cup, beat together the coconut oil, eggs, monk fruit, applesauce, and vanilla until well mixed, using the electric hand mixer.

4. Stir in the mixture of almond flour until well mixed, together with the blueberries. Let a batter stand for 5 minutes so the moisture can continue to be absorbed by the coconut flour.

5. Divide into 12 muffin cavities (use a large ice cream scoop for cooking the muffins with very domed tops) and bake until clean, approximately 24-25 minutes, golden brown, and insert a toothpick in the middle comes out.

6. Leave for 15 minutes to cool. Then, to remove them, loop a knife carefully along the sides of each muffin. Then, before attempting to take them out, let them cool perfectly in the pan.

2 Keto Zucchini Muffins With Almond Flour

Servings: 12 | **Time:** 30 mins | **Difficulty**: Easy

Nutrients per serving: Calories: 217 kcal | Fat: 18.5g | Carbohydrates: 8.6g | Protein: 8.2g | Fiber: 4g

Ingredients

1 1/2 Cups Monk fruit sweetener

1 Tbsp Ground Cardamom

1 Tbsp Ground cinnamon

1 tsp Baking soda

1 tsp Salt

1 tsp Vanilla extract

1/2 cup Tahini

2 Cups Grated zucchini, packed (about 2 medium zucchinis)

2 Large Eggs

2 tsp Baking powder

3 Cups Almond meal (10.5 oz)

5 Tbsp Unsweetened vanilla almond milk

Method

1. Preheat the oven to 350 F and adjust to one position below the oven rack center. Use cooking spray to spray a muffin pan.

2. Stir the almond meal, cardamom, baking powder, cinnamon, salt, and soda together in a medium bowl and set aside.

3. Using the electric hand mixer, mix the monk fruit, tahini, almond milk, eggs, and vanilla extract in a large bowl until well mixed.

4. The wet mixture adds the dry mixture and stirs until well mixed, and a thick batter emerges. Finally, fold in a grated zucchini softly when mixed uniformly.

5. Divide the mixture, filling up to the tip, into 12 muffin cavities. I like to use a huge scoop of ice cream, as it gives them a very good, domed top.

6. Bake for about 20-22 minutes, until a toothpick put in the middle, comes out clean. Let it cool for 10 minutes in the bath. Next, turn to a wire rack to cool off perfectly.

3 Sugar-Free Low Carb Keto Pecan Pie

Servings: 12 | **Time**: 1 day 55 mins | **Difficulty**: Easy

Nutrients per serving: Calories: 328.7 kcal | Fat: 31.1g | Carbohydrates: 18.8g | Protein: 5g | Fiber: 2.7g

Ingredients

6 Tbsp Unsalted butter

3/4 tsp Salt

2/3 cup Powdered erythritol sweetener (I used swerve)

2 large eggs

1 tsp Vanilla

1 tsp Maple extract

1 Almond flour pie crust

1 1/4 Cups Heavy whipping cream

1 1/2 Cups Pecans

Method

1. Whisk together all the sweetener and the butter in a big, high-sided frying pan set over medium- low heat. Cook, constantly whisking, until golden brown in the mixture, around 5-7 minutes.

2. When whisking continuously, throw in the creamy until golden and carry to a soft simmer.

3. Simmer, constantly stirring, around 8 minutes, until the mixture only starts to thicken. Remove from the heat and allow 30 minutes to cool.

4. Heat your oven to 350 F as it is cooling, then spread the pecans on the large baking sheet. Bake until browned and toasted for 10-12 minutes. Then, cut them loose and set them aside.

5. Add in eggs, salt, and the extracts and stir until smooth, until the mixture is cooled somewhat. Stir the pecans in.

6. Through the cooled pie crust, pour the filling and bake until the top feels firm, about 30 minutes. Let it cool at room temperature and cover overnight, and refrigerate.

7. Slice and devour the next day.

4 Low Carb Keto Mug Cake

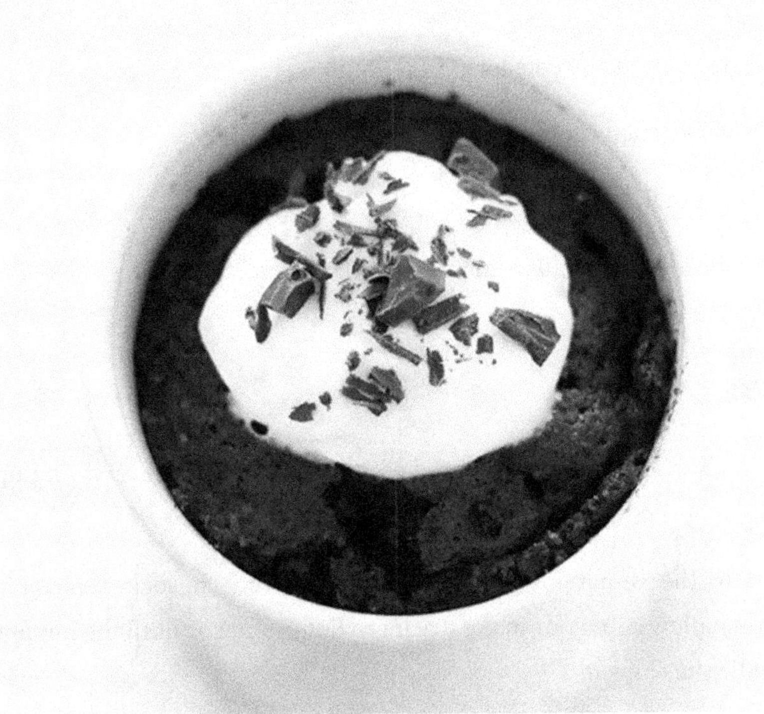

Servings: 1 | **Time:** 8 mins | **Difficulty**: Easy

Nutrients per serving: Calories: 312 kcal | Fat: 23.9g | Carbohydrates: 19.6g | Protein: 8.2g | Fiber: 11.6g

Ingredients

1 Egg yolk

1 Tbsp Coconut oil, melted

1 tsp Sugar-free chocolate chips

1/2 tsp Baking powder

1/2 tsp Vanilla extract

2 1/2 Tbsp Monkfruit sweetener

2 Tbsp Unsweetened cocoa powder

3 Tbsp Coconut flour

5 Tbsp Unsweetened vanilla almond milk Pinch of salt

Method

1. Whisk all of the dried ingredients in a small dish (everything up to the milk.)

2. Stir the remaining ingredients, minus the chocolate chips, in a separate, shallow cup. Pour in the dry ingredients and stir until the mixture is tender. Stir the chips in.

3. Transfer to a wide mug (14-16oz at least) and distributed evenly.

4. Cook it until the top is fixed and it is no bigger than a dime on some wet spots.

5 Keto Chocolate Peanut Butter Fat Bombs

Servings: 12 | **Time**: 1 hr 10 mins | **Difficulty:** Easy

Nutrients per serving: Calories: 127 kcal | Fat: 11.6g | Carbohydrates: 3.7g | Protein: 3.8g | Fiber: 1.4g

Ingredients

30-40 Drops Liquid stevia (to taste)

3/4 Cup Natural creamy peanut butter (may also use almond butter)

3 Tbsp cocoa powder (Unsweetened)

3 Tbsp Coconut oil

Method

1. Line a mini muffin tin with liners for mini muffins.

2. In a big, microwave-safe dish, put the coconut oil and peanut butter and heat until smooth and molten, for about 1 min.

3. Whisk in the powder with the chocolate until smooth. Then, to taste, whisk the stevia in.

4. Cover about 3/4 of the way, complete with the muffin cavities. Place the pan gently in the refrigerator and cool for around 1 hour, until solid.

6 Black Walnut Chocolate Chip Muffins With Almond Flour

Servings: 12 | **Time:** 40 mins | **Difficulty:** Easy

Nutrients per serving: Calories: 292 kcal | Fat: 26.1g | Carbohydrates: 10.9g | Protein: 8.3g | Fiber: 5.8g

Ingredients

1 Tbsp of Baking powder

1 Tbsp Vanilla extract

1 tsp of Baking soda

1/2 cup + 1 Tbsp Stevia-sweetened chocolate chips

1/4 Cup Hammons Black Walnuts, diced

3 cups Almond flour (300g)

3 large eggs, at room temperature (important)

3/4 cup of Monkfruit

1 tsp of Salt

4 Tbsp Coconut flour, firmly packed (32g)

6 Tbsp of Full-fat coconut milk (canned)

6 Tbsp of melted Ghee

Method

1. Preheat the oven to 350 °F and coat a muffin pan generously with cooking spray.

2. Mix the almond flour, baking powder, coconut flour, baking soda, and salt in a big dish.

3. Beat the monk fruit, coconut milk, eggs, ghee, and vanilla in a wide cup, using the electric hand mixer, until well mixed.

4. Add the mixture of flour and whisk until it is well mixed. Stir in the black walnuts and chocolate chips. It's going to be moist for your combination, much like cookie dough. Then sit for 5 mins so that the moisture can start to absorb the coconut flour.

5. Fill your muffin tin around 2/3 of the way (we like to use ice cream scoop to make the muffins look cool and domed) and bake on until tops are golden brown, about 25-27 minutes, and insert a toothpick in the middle comes out clean.

6. Let the cool pan Full. Then, loosen them with a knife along each muffin's edges and separate them from the tray.

7 Keto Pumpkin Cheesecake

Servings: 12 | **Time**: 2 hrs 20 mins | **Difficulty**: Easy

Nutrients per serving: Calories: 242 kcal | Fat: 23g | Carbohydrates: 5.7g | Protein: 6.5g | Fiber: 1.5g

Ingredients

3/4 cup Monkfruit

2/3 Cup Canned pumpkin

2 large eggs, at room temp

16 Oz Full fat cream cheese, at room temperature (2 blocks)

1 Tbsp Vanilla extract

1 Tbsp Pumpkin Pie Spice

1 Gluten-free Graham Cracker Crust, baked in a 9-inch springform pan

Method

1. Preheat up to 325 °F in your oven.

2. Beat the cream cheese and the monk fruit together in a large bowl using the electric hand mixer until smooth and well mixed.

3. Include all the ingredients, then beat until they are mixed. Don't beat it too hard, or the entrance of too much air in the cheesecake will cause it to sink during baking.

4. With 2 or 3 layers of tinfoil, take the graham cracker crust first from the freezer and then wrap the bottom and the sides very firmly. Place the pan in a large pan for roasting.

5. Onto the crust, pour the cheesecake, and smooth out uniformly. Switch to your oven's middle rack and cover the pan with water until the springform pan comes halfway up.

6. Bake for about 55-60 minutes, until the outside is set and a little circle in the middle is jiggly. Turn the oven off and gently break the lock, allowing the cheesecake to sit for 15 minutes in the oven. Shift to the counter to cool fully, then.

7. Cover up and refrigerate for 8 hours until cool, but better if overnight.

8. Hover a knife down the sides of a cheesecake softly, cut the pan and slice it out.

8 Sugar-Free No-Bake Keto Cheesecake

Servings: 2 | **Time:** 5 mins | **Difficulty**: Easy

Nutrients per serving: Calories: 292 kcal | Fat: 28g | Carbohydrates: 4.9g | Protein: 8g | Fiber: 0.9g

Ingredients

For The Crust:

1 tsp Powdered Erythritol Sweetener (I used Swerve)

2 tsp Ghee or butter, melted

3 Tbsp Almond flour, packed

The Cheesecake:

0.5 Cup Cream cheese (softened to room temperature)

0.5 tsp Vanilla extract

8-12 tsp of Powdered Erythritol Sweetener (to taste)

4 Tbsp 2% Plain Greek yogurt

Method

1. Stir the almond flour with sweetener together in a shallow dish. In the ghee, add in and mix until crumbly. Push a tiny ramekin onto the rim.

2. Beat a cream cheese plus sweetener in a medium bowl using the electric hand mixer. Add Cream cheese and vanilla, then beat until mixed again, keeping the sides from scraping as desired.

3. To taste sugar again. Spoon over crust and smoothly spread out. To firm up cream cheese, cool for at least 2 hours.

9 Sugar-Free Keto Lemon Bars

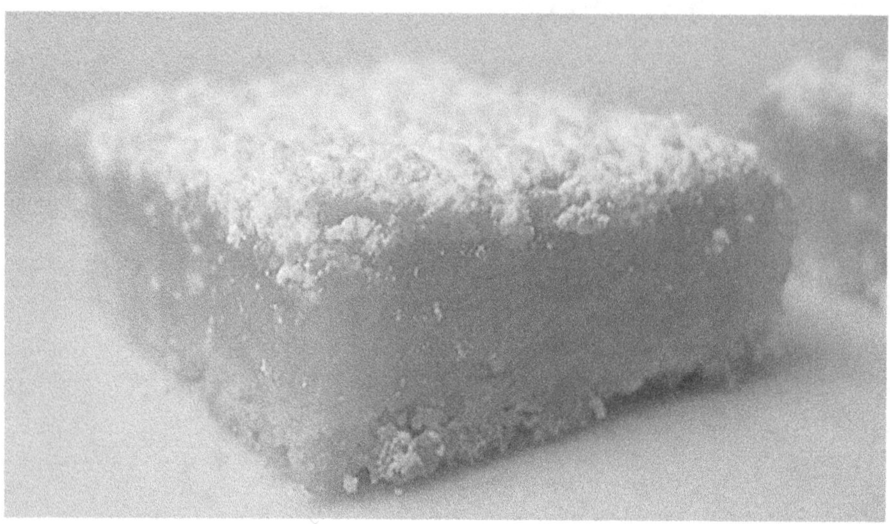

Servings: 16 | **Time:** 1 hr 25 mins | **Difficulty**: Easy

Nutrients per serving: Calories: 106 kcal | Fat: 8.9g | Carbohydrates: 4.7g | Protein: 2.5g | Fiber: 2.3g

Ingredients

For The Crust:

Pinch of salt

2 Tbsp Monkfruit

1/2 cup Coconut oil

1 cup of Coconut flour (95g)

For The Topping:

3/4 Cup Fresh lemon juice (about 6 large juicy lemons)

1 1/2 tsp Coconut flour, sifted

1/2 cup Monkfruit

2 tsp of Lemon zest

4 Eggs

Method

1. Preheat oven to 350 °F and use coconut oil to generously oil an 8x8 inch pan. Only put aside.

2. Include the coconut flour until it forms a dough.

3. Press the dough uniformly into the pan and bake for about 10 minutes, until just slightly golden brown.

4. Carefully stir together the lemon zest and eggs in a wide bowl until the crust has cooled.

10 Keto Brownies

Servings: 16 | **Time**: 30 mins | **Difficulty**: Easy

Nutrients per serving: Calories: 107 kcal | Fat: 10g | Carbohydrates: 5.7g | Protein: 2.5g | Fiber: 2.9g

Ingredients

1 large egg

1/2 tsp Baking soda

1/2 tsp Mint extract

1/4 cup Plant-based chocolate protein powder

1/4 tsp Sea salt

2 Egg yolks

2 Tbsp vanilla almond milk (Unsweetened)

5 ounces Sugar-free chocolate (roughly chopped and divided)

6 Tbsp Erythritol Sweetener

7 Tbsp Coconut oil (melted and divided)

Method

1. Preheat the oven to 350 °F and use coconut oil to generously oil an 8x8 inch pan. Put aside.

2. Beat the coconut oil and monk fruit and a pinch of salt together in a large bowl, using an electric hand mixer, until smooth and well mixed. Include coconut flour until it forms a dough.

3. Press the dough uniformly into the pan and bake for about 10 minutes, until just softly golden brown. Leave to cool for 30 minutes.

4. Lower the oven temperature to 325 ^{o}F and make sure that the oven rack is in the center of the oven.

5. Carefully stir together the lemon zest and eggs in a wide bowl until the crust has cooled. Don't use an electric blender here, or once fried, you can top with crack.

6. Heat the lemon juice softly in a separate, medium dish. Whisk in and stir in the monk fruit until it is dissolved. At room temperature, let it cool fully.

11 Peanut Butter Truffles

Servings: 10 Truffles | **Time:** 30 mins | **Difficulty:** Easy

Nutrients per serving (2 Truffles): Calories: 132 kcal | Fat: 9.9g | Carbohydrates: 10.9g | Protein: 4.4g | Fiber: 5.6g

Ingredients

2 tbsp Choc Zero Vanilla Syrup (Sugar-Free)

1/4 cup peanut butter

1/4 cup Coconut flour

1/3 cup chocolate chips (sugar-free)

Method

1. Mix all the peanut butter and the sugar-free syrup in a medium-sized dish.

2. To mix, add the coconut flour and mix. You are looking for a quality that you can roll into balls quickly. You can change the consistency if it is too moist or too dry by adding more coconut flour or the sweetener if required.

3. Take heaped Tsp. fuls of the blend and roll between your hands into balls. Move them to a plate or tray lined with paper that is oil proof.

4. Place the truffles for 10-20 minutes in the freezer until they are solid.

5. Melt the chocolate chips, meanwhile.

6. Take the truffles from the fridge and use the chocolate to decorate them. You should dip them in full or drizzle on top with a little chocolate-up it's to you.

7. For up to 1 week, you can store it in the refrigerator.

12 Creamy Keto Chia Pudding

Servings: 2 | **Time**: 6 hrs 10 mins | **Difficulty:** Easy

Nutrients per serving: Calories: 258 kcal | Fat: 18g | Carbohydrates: 8.15g | Protein: 3.66g | Fiber: 4.3g

Ingredients

1 cup Coconut milk full-fat

1 dash Salt

1/4 tsp Vanilla extract

1/4-1/2 tsp Stevia glycerite

2 tbsp Sugar-free jam

3 tbsp Black chia seeds

Method

1. In a small mug, mix the chia seeds and 1/2 cup of coconut milk.

2. Whisk together the vanilla, salt, and the leftover coconut milk. Use your preferred liquid sweetener to sweeten the flavor.

3. After 30 minutes, refrigerate and stir well to avoid Chia seeds from clumping at the bottom of the container. Overnight, refrigerate.

4. Layer the chia pudding in a serving cup or a small compact container of 1 Tbsp. of sugar-free jelly. Store in your refrigerator for up to 5 days.

13 Cranberry Almond Crumb Muffins

Servings: 12 | **Time:** 40 mins | **Difficulty**: Easy

Nutrients per serving: Calories: 330 kcal | Fat: 28.73g | Carbohydrates: 9.46g | Protein: 8.12g | Fiber: 5g

Ingredients

Dry Ingredients (divided use)

1/2 cup coconut flour (50 g)

1/2 cup low carb sugar (115 g)

1/2 Tsp. baking soda

1/2 Tsp. salt

1 1/2 cups fresh cranberries chopped, (115 g)

2 cups almond flour (185 g)

2 Tsp. baking powder

2 Tbsp. psyllium husk powder (20 gm)

Wet Ingredients

6 large eggs

1 Tsp. vanilla extract

1 Tbsp. white vinegar

1/2 Tsp. stevia glycerite

1/2 Tsp. almond extract

1/2 cup full-fat coconut milk (118 ml)

Crumb Mixture

1/4 cup sliced almonds a small handful

1/3 cup reserved dry ingredients (35 g)

2 Tbsp. low carb sugar

1 Tbsp. coconut oil melted (or butter)

Method

1. Preheat the oven to 350 °F and raise the lower third of the rack.

2. With the paper liners, line a muffin pan or brush well with the baking spray. °F

3. Dry Ingredients: Weigh into a medium bowl the first 6 ingredients - NOT the psyllium husk powder.

4. To break up any lumps and to spread the ingredients equally, whisk well.

5. Drop 1/3 cup of the dry mixture and place it in a small dish.

6. To add the muffin ingredients, add the psyllium husk powder and stir again.

7. On top, pour the chopped cranberries.

8. If the tops are well browned, insert a toothpick into the center of a muffin comes out clean, and the cranberry muffins are finished.

14 Buttery Keto Pecan Sandies Cookies

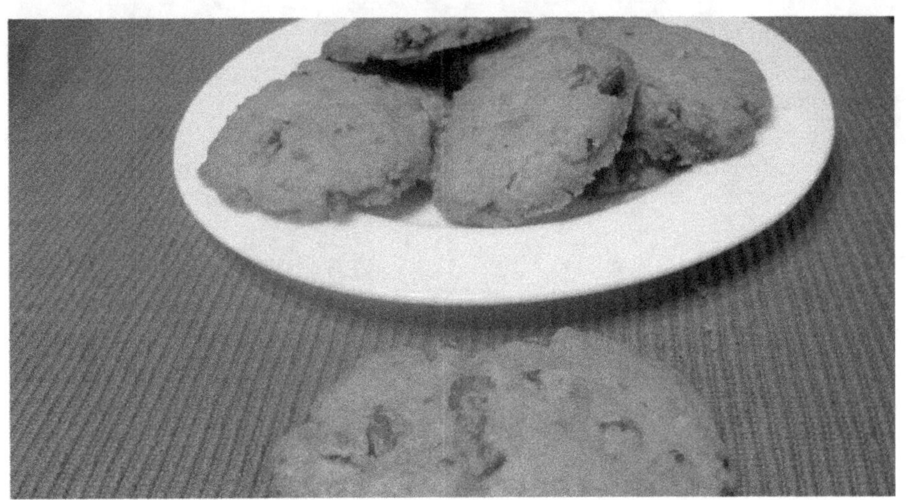

Servings: 18 cookies | **Time:** 1 hr 22 mins | **Difficulty:** Easy

Nutrients per serving: Calories: 126 kcal | Fat: 12.16g | Carbohydrates: 3.2g | Protein: 2.33g | Fiber: 2.4g

Ingredients

1 1/2 tsp Xanthan gum

1 cup Almond flour (90 g)

1 cup Pecans (4 oz/ 113 g)

1 Egg white beaten

1 tsp Vanilla

1/2 cup Low carb sugar (90 g)

1/2 cup Oat fiber (34 g)

1/4 tsp Baking soda

2 tsp Gelatin (optional)

8 tbsp cold salted butter cut into small pieces

Extra sweetener for dipping tops (2 tbsp)

Method

1. Preheat the oven to 350 and place the rack in the center position. Using parchment paper to cover a sheet pan.

2. Pour pecans and cut them into tiny pieces in the food processor.

3. To combine, add the next Six ingredients and mix.

4. Cut butter into the small pieces and add it until put into the food processor, grinding.

5. Beat vanilla into the white egg in a tiny cup.

6. The food processor spread the mixture equally all around ingredients and pulse until the dough is uniformly moist.

15 Keto Cranberry Crumb Bars

Servings: 16 | **Time:** 1 hr | **Difficulty**: Easy

Nutrients per serving: Calories: 196 kcal | Fat: 14g | Carbohydrates: 8g| Protein: 4g | Fiber: 3g

Ingredients

Cranberry Filling

1 cup water (236.58 g)

1 pinch fresh ground nutmeg

1 pinch salt

1 Tbsp. lemon juice (15 ml) or 3 Real Lemon packets

1/2 cup low carbohydrates powdered sugar (80 g)

12 ounces cranberries (340 g) fresh or frozen Shortbread Crust

2 cups almond flour (180 g)

1 cup shredded coconut (90 g) ground in a coffee grinder

1/3 cup whey protein powder (20 g)

1/3 cup low carb powdered sugar (50 g)

1/2 Tsp. salt

8 Tbsp. salted butter melted Crumb Topping

3/4 cup of a shortbread crust mixture

1/2 cup chopped walnuts (40 g)

3 Tbsp. Low carb brown sugar (35 g)

3 Tbsp. Sugar-Free Chocolate Chips (40 g)

Method

1. By cutting a parchment's strips large enough to fill the pan's bottom and go up to two respective ends and hangover, prepare an 8x8 or 9x9 brownie pan.

2. With baking spray, spray the pan and placed the piece of parchment in the pan, smoothing it to match. Then you have to chop the walnuts.

3. Place all of the cranberry filling ingredients in a medium pot and bring it to a boil.

4. For 10-15 minutes, simmer gently until a mixture thickens.

5. When the cranberries are frying, process the crushed coconut until it is finely ground in a coffee grinder or small food processor.

6. In a medium dish, place all the dry ingredients for a shortbread crust.

7. The butter is warmed and poured over the dry ingredients.

16 Low Carb Apple Crumb Muffins

Servings: 12 | **Time:** 45 mins | **Difficulty**: Easy

Nutrients per serving: Calories: 155 kcal | Fat: 12g | Carbohydrates: 9g | Protein: 5.86g | Fiber: 5.6g

Ingredients

Dry Ingredients (divided use)

2 cups Almond flour (190 g)

2 tsp Baking powder

1/2 cup Oat fiber (45 g)

1/2 cup Low Carb Brown Sugar (80 g)

1/2 tsp Baking soda

1/2 tsp Xanthan gum

1/2 tsp ground cardamom

1/4 tsp Allspice

1/4 tsp ground ginger

1/4 tsp Salt

Wet Ingredients

4 large Eggs

1 tsp Vanilla extract

1/2 tsp Stevia glycerite

2/3 cup Coconut milk (full fat)(158 ml)

3/4 large Granny Smith apple peeled, cored, and grated

(5 oz/ 141 g) Crumb Topping

1/3 cup of dry ingredients

1 tbsp of melted butter (ghee or coconut oil)

1 tbsp Granulated erythritol

Method

1. Preheat Oven to 325 °F. Line up the 12 cup muffin tin with the baking paper of the usual size.

2. Peel the Granny Smith apple.

3. Weigh 5 ounces and grate them (about 3/4 of a big apple).

4. In a medium cup, weigh all the dry ingredients and blend them to break up the lumps.

5. To use as the crumb topping, stir 1/3 cup of a mixture into a small dish.

6. Fill a large bowl with all the grated apple and wet ingredients.

7. Blend with the hand mixer.

8. Pour dry ingredients into wet ingredients and mix until they are combined.

17 Coconut Flour Chocolate Chip Cookies

Servings: 8 | **Time:** 20 mins | **Difficulty**: Easy

Nutrients per serving: Calories: 71 kcal | Fat: 6.44g | Carbohydrates: 2.85g | Protein: 1.31g | Fiber: 2g

Ingredients

2 tbsp Low carb brown sugar (or your favorite granulated sweetener)

2 tbsp Light Olive Oil

2 tbsp Almond Butter or nut/seed butter of choice

1/4 cup Coconut Flour

1/2 tsp Vanilla Extract

1 tbsp Lily's Sugar-Free Chocolate Chips or 85-90% dark chocolate

1 tbsp Flax Meal

1 pinch Salt

Method

1. In a medium mixing cup, prepare the flax egg by stirring 1 tbsp of flax meal and 2.5 tbsp of water together. To thicken, leave for a few minutes.

2. Using a spatula, whisk in the vanilla extract and almond butter, and sunflower oil.

3. Add low-carb brown sugar, a touch of salt, and coconut flour to taste. To shape the dough, blend well.

4. Stir in the chips or bits of chocolate. Take 1 Tbsp. of cookie dough and roll your hands into a ball. Place the ball and flatten it into a cookie shape on a baking tray (the cookies will not spread - thinner cookies result in a crisper cookie).

5. Repeat for the cookie dough that remains.

6. At 350 F/ 180 C or until crispy around the outside, bake the cookies for about 15 minutes. Don't bake over them. Enjoy when fully refrigerated.

7. Store in the refrigerator in an airtight jar. Refrigerating mitigates the erythritol-based sweetener's cooling feeling.

18 Keto Chocolate Chia Pudding

Servings: 2 | **Time**: 35 mins | **Difficulty:** Easy

Nutrients per serving: Calories: 336 kcal | Fat: 27.3g | Carbohydrates: 16g | Protein: 8g | Fiber: 11g

Ingredients

2 tbsp low carb sugar (Sukrin:1, Swerve, Lakanto, Truvia, or Besti)

1 tsp Vanilla Extract

1 tbsp Cocoa Powder (sift before measuring)

1 cup Coconut Milk (from a can) (or Almond Milk for fewer calories)

1/4 cup Chia Seeds

Method

1. To a mason jar, apply the chocolate powder and sweetener. To clear some lumps, shake well.

2. To the mason jar, apply vanilla extract and coconut milk. tIn order to mix, close the lid, and then shake.

3. Apply to the jar the chia seeds and shake again. Move the container to the fridge until the mixture is well mixed.

4. For at least 30 min, cool it.

5. Serve a chocolate chia pudding with almond yogurt and seasonal fruit in your favorite jars.

19 Fluffy Keto Banana Cream Pie

Servings: 8 | **Time:** 55 mins | **Difficulty:** Easy

Nutrients per serving: Calories: 526 kcal | Fat: 47g | Carbohydrates: 9.8g | Protein: 11g | Fiber: 4.3g

Ingredients

Low Carb Crust

1 recipe Low Carbohydrates Walnut Pie Crust Banana Pudding (refrigerate overnight)

1 cup heavy cream

1 tbsp arrowroot powder

1 pinch salt

3 large egg yolks

2 large eggs

2 tbsp butter

1 tsp vanilla

1 tsp banana extract

1/2 cup low carb sugar (Swerve granulated or Lakanto)

1/3 cup almond milk

1 1/4 tsp gelatin powder

1/8 tsp xanthan gum

Whipped Cream (for folding into the Banana pudding)

2 tbsp low carb powdered sugar (or Swerve Confection or Lakanto Powdered)

1/8 tsp xanthan gum

1/2 cup heavy cream

Method

1. 1.Make the Low Carbohydrate Walnut Pie Crust according to the direction. Make it cool.

2. Ready by the stove for a strainer. To bloom, spray the gelatin over 1 Tbsp. of water.

3. In a medium saucepan, put the cream & almond milk, turn heat to medium before the milk steams, and create bubbles across the pan sides.

4. Whisk the arrowroot, sweetener, xanthan gum, and salt together in a medium dish. To mix, add the egg yolks or whole eggs and whisk.

5. Add the hot milk into the egg mixture in a thin stream while constantly whisking.

20 Low Carb Lemon Curd

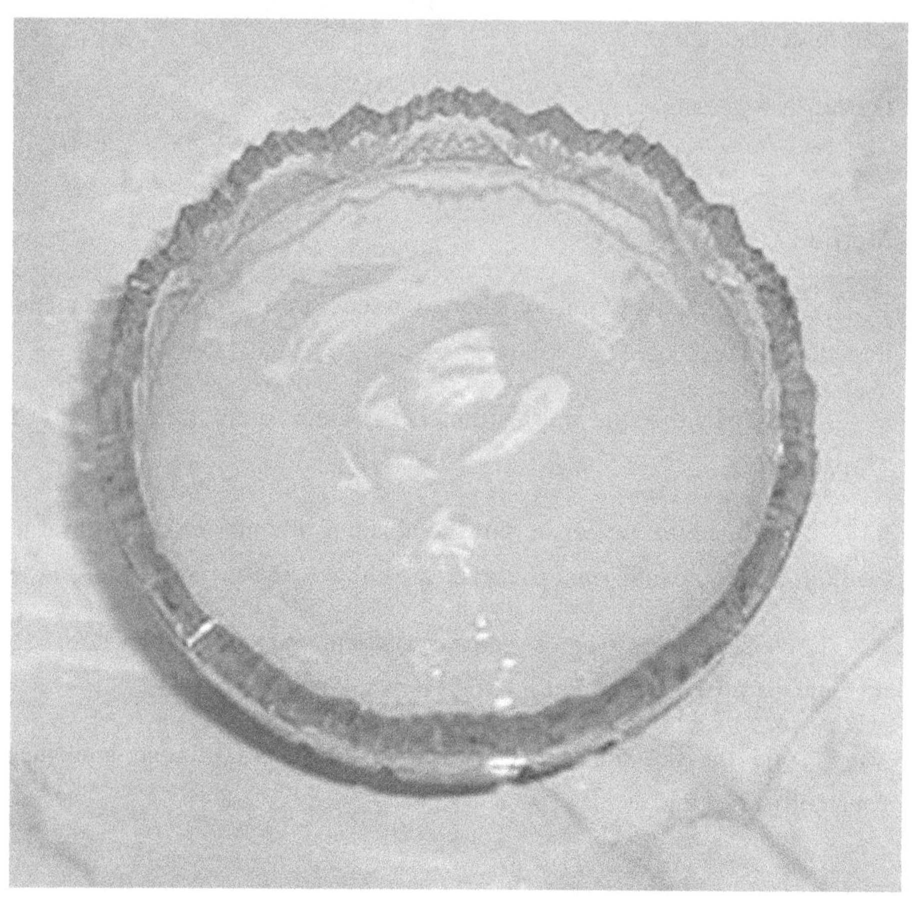

Servings: 10 | **Time:** 25 mins | **Difficulty:** Easy

Nutrients per serving: Calories: 120 kcal | Fat: 10.7g | Carbohydrates: 2.6g | Protein: 3.74g | Fiber: 0.1g

Ingredients

3/4 cup (6 ounces) lemon juice, about 3-4 large lemons

1/4 Tsp. stevia glycerite

1/2 cup low carb sugar (or Swerve, or Lakanto Monkfruit)

4 large eggs

4 large egg yolks

the zest from all of the lemons

6 Tbsp. salted butter

1 Tbsp. arrowroot powder

Method

1. Weigh and put the erythritol and the arrowroot powder in a medium bath. Stir it together.

2. To make them juicy, roll the lemons on the table, then zest the lemons, applying the zest to erythritol.

3. Separate four eggs and apply the yolks to the pot of erythritol.

4. To the bowl, add the 4 whole eggs and whisk together the eggs and erythritol.

5. Juice and weigh 3/4 cup of the lemons.

6. Strain the juice from the lemon and whisk it into the eggs.

7. Down to medium-low, switch the heat, and finish whisking.

21 Low Carb Lemon Lush Dessert

Servings: 15 | **Time:** 9 hrs 30 mins | **Difficulty**: Easy

Nutrients per serving: Calories: 308 kcal | Fat: 29g | Carbohydrates: 6.4g | Protein: 7g | Fiber: 1.9g

Ingredients

Lemon Curd (time: 20 minutes)

1 recipe Lemon Curd (chilled at least 4 hours)

Shortbread Crust (time: 30 minutes) (cool completely)

3/4 cup pecans, finely chopped

1/3 cup whey protein powder

1/3 cup of powdered sweetener (Swerve, Sukrin, or Lakanto)

2 cups almond flour

7 tbsp of salted butter (melted)

Cream Cheese Layers (time: 10 minutes)

1 tsp vanilla extract

1/4 cup heavy whipping cream (2 fl oz)

1/4 cup powdered sweetener (Sukrin, Swerve, or Lakanto)

16 oz softened cream cheese (2 packages)

Heavy whipping cream (divided use) (time: 10 minutes)

2 cups heavy whipping cream

2 tbsp powdered sweetener

1 tsp vanilla

1/8 tsp xanthan gum (optional - stabilizes the whipped cream) Assembly (about 10 minutes)

Method

1. Before assembling the cake, prepare a lemon curd and allow it to cool fully for about 4 hours. It is possible to do this many days in advance. It is also excellent to make the shortbread crust ahead.

Pecan Shortbread Crust

1. Preheat the oven to 350 °F. Chop the pecans fairly fine and mix in a small bowl with the rest of the dry ingredients. To mix, whisk together. Melt the butter and pour the spices over it. To form a sticky, crumbly paste, combine with a fork.

2. Pour the materials into a pyrex baking dish of 13x9 inch glass and lay a waxed paper layer on the mixture. Use both fingertips, and press tightly into the bottom of a pan with a flat bottom bottle or measurement cup. Remove a waxed paper, then bake for about 15 minutes, until softly golden.

Whipped Cream

Whip the vanilla and sweeteners with the milk until it is stiff.

Cream Cheese Layer

Whip the cream cheese until nice and light with 1/4 of heavy cream and a sweetener. Adding 1/2 cup of whipped cream at a time, fold 1 1/2 cups of the whipped cream into the cream cheese. Over a shortbread crust, spread evenly.

Lemon Curd Layer

1. When loosened, whisk the lemon curd and scatter softly over the cream cheese surface. Spread the leftover whipped cream gently over the lemon curd. It is better to refrigerate for several hours or overnight.

22 Sugar-Free Pecan Turtle Cheesecake Bars

Servings: 16 | **Time:** 30 mins | **Difficulty**: Easy

Nutrients per serving: Calories: 439 kcal | Fat: 42g | Carbohydrates: 13g | Protein: 6g | Fiber: 8g

Ingredients

1 recipe Homemade Low Carbohydrates Caramel Sauce

1 recipe Low Carbohydrates

Hot Fudge Sauce

Brown Sugar Pecan Crust

4 Tbsp. salted butter, (melted) (2 oz/ 57 g)

1/4 cup of whey protein powder (25 g)

1/3 cup of Sukrin Gold powdered (70 g)

1 cup toasted pecans, (ground) (4 oz/ 114 g)

1 cup of Almond Flour (4 oz / 114 g)

Vanilla Cheesecake

1 Tbsp. (15 g) vanilla extract

2 1/2 packages cream cheese, (softened) (20 oz / 567 g)

1/2 cup heavy cream, (whipped) (4 oz/ 118.29 ml)

1/2 Tsp. of Stevia Glycerite

2/3 cup of low carb powdered sugar (3 oz / 85 g)

Topping

fudge sauce for drizzling caramel

sauce for drizzling

1 cup toasted pecans, chopped (4 oz/ 114 g)

Method

1. Preheat the oven to 350 F and toast the pecans all.

2. Spray a 9X9 inch wide baking pan with baking spray and cover with a long enough parchment sheet such that two sides hang over it.

3. This will allow you to remove the bars for faster cutting and to serve in 1 big section.

4. 4.Grind the Sukrin Gold and add it to a medium bowl in a coffee grinder.

5. In a coffee grinder, grind the pecans and apply the sweetener to the medium dish.

6. Apply the remainder of the dry ingredients and thoroughly mix.

7. Melt and blend the butter into the dry ingredients.

8. When pressed softly in your palm, the mixture should stay together. In the microwave, heat the caramel and hot fudge sauces until soft and stir with a pour-able consistency.

23 Keto Sour Cream Cake

Servings: 12 | **Time:** 50 mins | **Difficulty**: Easy

Nutrients per serving: Calories: 358 kcal | Fat: 34.5g | Carbohydrates: 7g | Protein: 8.6g | Fiber: 2.5g

Ingredients

Cake:

3 cups almond flour (280 g)

1 tsp sea salt

3 large eggs (I always use cold)

2 tsp vanilla extract

1/2 tsp baking soda

1/2 cup sour cream

1/2 tsp stevia glycerite

1/4 cup salted butter, melted (4 tbsp, 2 oz)

2/3 cup low carb sugar

Frosting:

6 oz cold cream cheese

3/4 cup heavy cream

1/4 tsp stevia glycerite

1/4 cup salted butter (very soft) (4 tbsp, 2 oz)

1/3 cup low carb powdered sugar

1 tsp vanilla extract

Garnish:

12 mint sprigs

36 small blueberries

6 medium strawberries, halved

Method

1. Preheat the oven to 350 F and place the rack in the center position. Spray a 1/4-sheet tray with baking spray (small jelly roll pan).

2. With parchment paper, line the bottom and spray a paper. Whisk the almond flour to break up some lumps before weighing with a whisk.

3. Measure into a medium-large bowl all the dry ingredients. Whisk to mix thoroughly. Add all the wet ingredients to dry ingredients and combine using a hand mixer thoroughly.

4. For the best results, spread the dense batter onto the ready sheet pan and smooth uniformly with an offset spatula.

5. Bake for 20-30 minutes. When gently pressed with a finger, the cake must spring back but still sound mildly moist. Remove from the oven and perfectly cool.

6. Place a cold cream cheese with the vanilla extract, powdered sweetener, and stevia glycerite in a small-medium cup.

7. Beat until the cream cheese is fully smooth and soft with a hand mixer, around 1-2 min, scraping down each side to remove any leftover lumps.

24 Keto Chocolate Mug Cake

Servings: 1 | **Time**: 3 mins | **Difficulty:** Easy

Nutrients per serving: Calories: 272 kcal | Fat: 23g | Carbohydrates: 7g | Protein: 9g | Fiber: 4g

Ingredients

1 large egg yolk

1 tbsp cocoa powder

1 tbsp low carb sugar (Lakanto or Swerve)

1 tbsp mayonnaise (use sour cream in a pinch)

1 tsp water

1/4 tsp baking powder

2 tbsp almond flour

Method

a. Until weighing, fluff up the almond flour with a whisk and sift before measuring the cocoa powder.

b. Measure into a mug or jelly jar the dry ingredients and blend fully with a fork.

c. Add the egg yolk, mayonnaise, and water, stirring thoroughly to make sure you have all from the bottom. Leave the batter to rest for 1-2 minutes. Depending on the microwave, microwave for 50 seconds.

25 Lemon Ricotta Cake

Servings: 9 | **Time:** 1 hr | **Difficulty:** Easy

Nutrients per serving: Calories: 212 kcal | Fat: 17g | Carbohydrates: 7g | Protein: 8g | Fiber: 3.5g

Ingredients

1/2 stick soft butter (2 oz/57 g)

1/2 cup low carb sugar (Swerve Granulated or Lakanto Classic)

1 1/2 tbsp fresh lemon juice

4 large eggs (cold) (one more egg if not using baking powder)

1 cup whole milk ricotta cheese (cold) (250 g)

1 tsp lemon zest (zest from one lemon)

1 tsp vanilla extract

Dry Ingredients

1 cup almond flour (whisk before measuring)

1/4 tsp salt

2 tsp baking powder

4 tbsp coconut flour (whisk before measuring)

Method

1. To 325 °F. Preheat oven. To suit the inner bottom of an 8 x 2-inch circular pan, cut a slice of parchment. The pan is sprayed or buttered, and the parchment is applied.

2. In a small dish, weigh the dry ingredients and whisk to remove any lumps—the cream when fully mixed with the butter, vanilla, and sweetener.

3. Add one egg and beat until fluffy and light. Stir in the ricotta cheese, lemon zest, lemon juice, and beat until well mixed.

4. Mix 1/3 of the dry ingredients into the batter by working by thirds.

5. Add the egg and blend. Repeat by starting with the last egg with the remaining ingredients. Carefully spread the batter with an offset spatula into the prepared cake tray.

6. Bake for 50 minutes or until the middle of the cake comes out clean with a toothpick inserted. Wrap every remaining cake in cling film and leave for 3 days (unless it is hot and humid) or refrigerate in the fridge.

7. Slightly warm before eating, if refrigerated.

26 Keto Strawberry Crepes

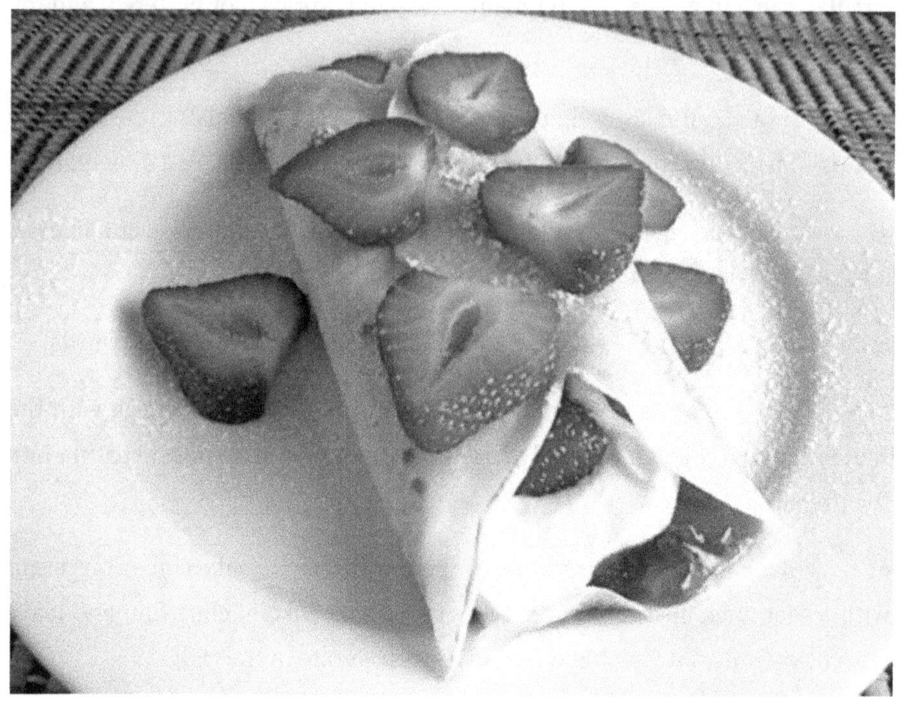

Servings: 4 | **Time**: 15 mins | **Difficulty:** Easy

Nutrients per serving: Calories: 316 kcal | Fat: 29g | Carbohydrates: 5g | Protein: 9g | Fiber: 0.5g

Ingredients

4 low carb crepes

4 tbsp low carb sugar (divided use)

3 ounces fresh strawberries, quartered and sliced

2 tsp Brandy, Rum, or Bourbon (optional, replace with water)

2 tsp water

1/2 cup Heavy Whipping Cream

1/2 tsp vanilla extract

1/2 cup sour cream

Method

1. In a small bowl with 1 tbsp of the sweetener, apply the brandy and water, and combine to dissolve. It does not completely dissolve. Slice the strawberries, then put them in a small dish. Apply the combination of brandy and stir. Put the bowl aside as you macerate the strawberries.

2. In a 2-3 cup mug, weigh the heavy cream, the leftover sweetener, and vanilla. Whip until very rigid.

3. In a shallow dish, apply the sour cream and whisk it to loosen. Spoon 1/4 of whipped cream onto the sour cream and mix the cream softly. Fold half of the leftover whipped cream with a large spoon or rubber spatula onto the sour cream mixture. Apply to the sour cream mixture the leftover whipped cream and fold together fully. (At this point, the filling could be refrigerated for up to a day.) (Makes around 1 1/2 cups)

4. Place half of each crepe with 1/4 of a whipped cream mixture, spreading just half of each crepe. Fold the exposed half over the filled side, then fold, like a handkerchief, corner to corner. On each tray, position one. (If sealed and refrigerated, the crepes should be filled for many hours before serving.)

5. Whisk the strawberries over each loaded crepe and spoon 1/4 of strawberries and juice on them. Serve.

27 Hazelnut Creme Brulee

Servings: 2 | **Time:** 40 mins | **Difficulty**: Easy

Nutrients per serving: Calories: 534 kcal | Fat: 52g | Carbohydrates: 4g | Protein: 7g

Ingredients

3 large egg yolks

2 tbsp spiced rum, brandy, or bourbon

2 tbsp low carb sugar (or Swerve Granular) (sugar, for non-low carbers)

1/4 tsp hazelnut extract

1 pinch salt

1 cup heavy cream

Optional (powdered sweetener for the top):

4 tsp Low carb brown sugar

Method

1. Preheat the oven to 350 °F and place the rack in the center position. Heat water until hot, not boiling, in a tea kettle. Halfway up the side of the ramekins, find a pan wide enough to accommodate 2, 6-oz ramekins and shallow enough to add water.

2. Add to a small bowl the yolks, and sweetener. With a fork, beat well to perfectly break up the yolks. Drop some giant chalazae.

3. In a small pot, pour the heavy cream and put it over medium heat. Stir with a whisk periodically before bubbles appear along the pot's edge, and the cream steams. Turn the heat off and start pouring the egg yolk into the mixture of the hot cream - very gently, in a thin stream, all the while whisking rapidly. Spiced rum (bourbon, brandy) and hazelnut extract are whisked in.

4. Divide the combination of creme brulee equally between the ramekins. Put the ramekins in the pan and fill the cooking pan with hot water halfway up the ramekin's sides (not boiling). Place the pan carefully in the oven and bake for thirty min or until the creme brulee is only centered in the very middle. (Depending on the form of the ramekin.o, it may always be just a little bit wiggly in the middle

5. In the water bath, cool the hazelnut creme brulee for 30 minutes before transferring it to a rack to cool entirely. Cover and refrigerate for about 4 hours with plastic wrap, but it's best overnight.

6. Sprinkle 1 tsp sweetener or over the tops of each creme brulee before serving. Melt the sweetener until it caramelizes, turning brown with a culinary torch. Instead, add to the top a dollop of whipped cream. Serve.

28 Sugar-Free Chocolate Pie

Servings: 10 | **Time**: 40 mins | **Difficulty**: Easy

Nutrients per serving: Calories: 337 kcal | Fat: 34g | Carbohydrates: 8g | Protein: 6g | Fiber: 5g

Ingredients

Flaky Pie Crust

5 tbsp butter

3 tbsp oat fiber

1/4 tsp salt

1 tsp water

1 large egg white

1 1/2 cup almond flour

Filling:

4 ounces unsweetened baking chocolate squares, melted

4 large pasteurized eggs, cold

2 Tsp. vanilla extract

6 ounces (1 1/2 sticks) salted butter, very soft

1/2 Tsp. stevia glycerite (or more Sukrin or Swerve to taste)

1 1/4 cups low carb powdered sugar (or Swerve Confectioners) 1/4 cup heavy cream

Topping:

chocolate shavings optional - I used 2 squares of Chocolate at 86% cacao

3/4 cup heavy cream

2 tbsp low carb powdered sugar (or swerve)

Method

1. Preheat the oven to 350°F. Using baking spray to spray a pie dish. I'm using a pyrex 9-inch baking dish. (On the pie plate base, we scatter sesame seeds, so the crust should not adhere to the bottom.)

2. Measure into the food processor the oat fiber, almond flour, and salt. Cut the butter into pellets and pulse with dry ingredients until the small peas are the butter's size. Mix 1 Tsp. of water with the white egg and spill over the dry ingredients. The phase before it all comes along with the dough. For about 30 minutes to 5 days, you can refrigerate the dough.

3. For your pie plate, roll the pastry into two sheets of plastic wrap until it becomes the right size. Remove the plastic top piece and invert dough over the plate of the pie. Coax the dough softly onto the bottom and sides of a plate. Remove the plastic and bring the edge into shape. With a fork, dock the dough.

4. Bake the crust for 10-15 minutes before the golden brown starts to transform. Let it cool fully, then cover until ready to use with plastic wrap.

5. Unsweetened baking chocolate is finely diced and stored in a microwaveable dish. Heat up to 30 secs at a time before it nearly melts. The excess heat from a bowl should ensure that the remainder is dissolved.

6. In a stand mixer or a large mixing cup, place the butter and Swerve or Sukrin Melis. Apply the paddle attachment to the mixer, then beat the

butter and a sweetener for around 2 minutes at medium speed. Give the bowl a scrape. Add the chocolate to the molten one and blend for 1 minute. Scrape thoroughly down the bowl. Apply 1/4 cup of heavy cream, vanilla, then glycerin stevia, and beat for 2 more minutes. Spread a filling back into a bowl and drop the paddle attachment.

7. Add the whisk attachment and switch back at medium speed on the stand mixer. Add one egg on time and let the mixer run between each addition for about 3 minutes, scraping the pan after the third and fourth additions.

8. Finish blending at high speed with a fast burst and disperse the filling into the pie's shell and refrigerate. [NOTE: refrigerate for 40 minutes if the filling splits (separates), then add 1/4 tsp of xanthan gum. Whip to release the filling for a few seconds at medium speed and then at high just a few seconds before it comes together. There could be another pinch of xanthan gum if required.]

9. With a spoon or spatula, spoon the filling onto the pie crust, then smooth it. Refrigerate, and leave open for 6 hours or overnight.

10. Whip the 3/4 cup heavy cream and finish the pie with your preferred sweetener. Additionally, by running the vegetable peeler down of a chocolate slice, chocolate curls may be added.

29 Sugar-free Nutella Swirl Muffins

Servings: 6 | **Time**: 40 mins | **Difficulty**: Easy

Nutrients per serving: Calories: 255 kcal | Fat: 22g | Carbohydrates: 6g | Protein: 9g | Fiber: 1g

Ingredients

Dry Ingredients

1/4 tsp salt

1 tsp baking powder

1 tbsp whey protein powder (We use Isopure Zero Carb)

1 1/2 cups Almond Flour (130 g)

Wet Ingredients

2 large eggs

1/2 cup heavy cream

1 1/2 tsp vanilla extract

1/3 cup low carb sugar

Swirl Topping

6 tsp Free Chocolate Hazelnut Spread (Sukrin Sugar)

Method

1. Preheat the oven to 350 F and put the rack in the center position. Strip 6 muffin wells of standard size with parchment liners. In the microwave, heat a Sukrin Chocolate Hazelnut Spread for 20-30 seconds or until a Tsp. is easy to drizzle.

2. Place the wet ingredients in the mixer. Place the dry ingredients in the mixer then. Switch down the mixer and mix. With a spatula, cut the lid and help the phase-out. Turn to medium-low and mix for 20 seconds just until the batter is smooth and well ventilated.

3. Divide the muffin batter, filling 3/4 full, among six muffin wells. Drizzle 1 Tsp. of Sukrin Chocolate Hazelnut Spread and swirl/mix with a toothpick over each muffin.

4. Bake for about 25-35 minutes or until the muffin tops are smooth to the touch and springy but still sound moist. Cool in the muffin tin for 5 minutes, then remove from a cooling rack. Refrigerate for 7-10 days in an airtight jar or stock for up to 5 days on the fridge.

30 Moist Chocolate Walnut Cake

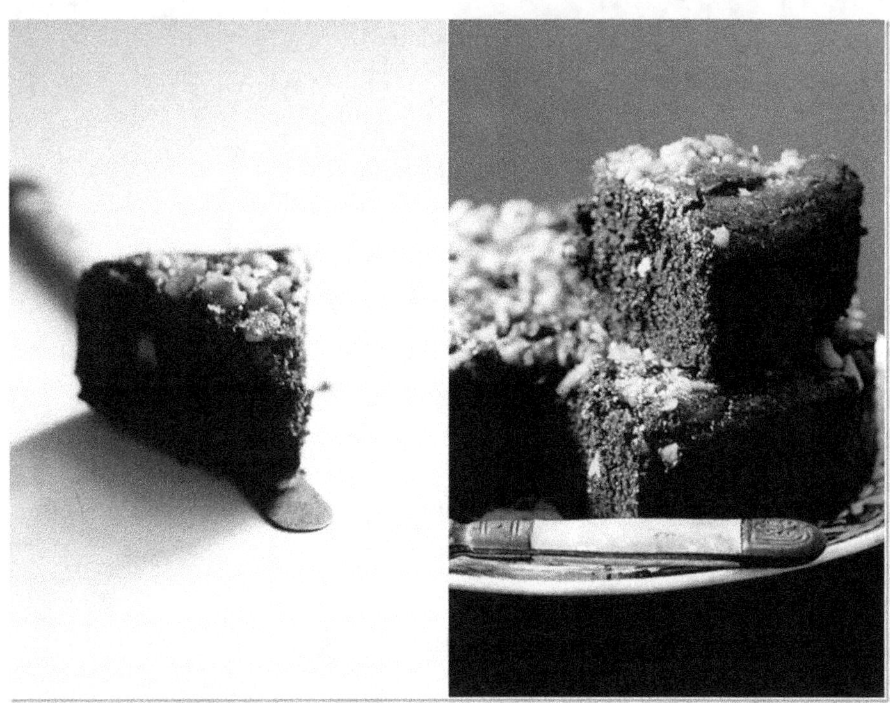

Servings: 12 | **Time**: 55 mins | **Difficulty**: Easy

Nutrients per serving: Calories: 264 kcal | Fat: 23g | Carbohydrates: 10g | Protein: 8g | Fiber: 5g

Ingredients

Dry Ingredients

3 ounces walnuts

1/4 Tsp. salt

1/3 cup coconut flour (fluff up with whisk before measuring)

1/3 cup cocoa powder (sift then measure)

1/2 cup low carb sugar (or Swerve Granulated)

1 tbsp baking powder

1 1/4 cup almond flour (whisk before measuring)

Wet Ingredients

4 large eggs

1 Tsp. vanilla

1 Tsp. stevia glycerite

1/2 cup buttermilk (or heavy cream or full-fat coconut milk)

1/4 cup walnut oil (or melted butter)

Chocolate Ganache Glaze

1/4 cup heavy cream

2 oz Ghiradelli Intense Dark Chocolate (86% or any high percentage chocolate)

2 Tbsp. butter or coconut oil (room temperature)

Method

a. Preheat the oven to 325 °F and put the rack in the center of the oven. On the sheet of waxed paper or the parchment, trace the base of an 8 x 2 inches cake tray. Cut the circle out. Spray the cake pan with the baking spray and line the parchment circle at the pan's bottom. Weigh the walnuts and grind the sweetener until finely ground in a food processor.

b. In a medium cup, weigh the dry cake ingredients (along with ground walnuts) and vigorously stir with a large whisk to mix. Add the wet ingredients to another bowl and pound them with a hand mixer. Add the wet ingredients to the dry dish and combine until all the ingredients are thoroughly integrated.

c. To dislodge some large air bubbles, spoon the batter in the cake pan and softly tap it on a counter 2-3 times. When carefully squeezed with your finger and insert a toothpick in the middle, bake for about 30-40 minutes or until the cake still looks moist. Do not bake in excess.

d. Take a Chocolate Walnut Cake from the oven and cover it with a clean tea towel. Let the cake perfectly cold. Then seal until ready to cover with ganache in plastic wrap. Until topping with the ganache, ensure that the cake is at room temperature.

e. Finely cut the chocolate and put it with the heavy cream and butter in a shallow microwaveable dish. Cover with waxed paper, then microwave for 30 seconds. For 1 minute, let stand, then gently whisk to mix. The ganache should be rich and shiny. Use it instantly.

f. Pour a chocolate ganache in the middle of a cake and spread it over the side with a spatula or knife, causing it to spill. Decorate, if you wish, with walnut halves (optional) or pieces of walnut while the ganache is still moist. Once the ganache has set, cut, and serve (it will still be fairly soft but not runny).

g. Hold it in the fridge or on the table. Let it arrive at room temperature for about 30 minutes before having it if refrigerated.

31 Blackberry Custard Pie

Servings: 10 | **Time:** 20 mins | **Difficulty:** Easy

Nutrients per serving: Calories: 357 kcal | Fat: 32g | Carbohydrates: 8g | Protein: 11g | Fiber: 3g

Ingredients

4 large eggs

3/4 cup heavy cream

2 large egg yolks

1/4 tsp xanthan gum

1/2 cup low carb sugar

1 tsp vanilla extract

1 tsp gelatin powder (flourished in 1 tbsp water)

1 recipe Low Carbohydrates Keto Graham Cracker Crust (resists soaking)

1 pinch salt

1 pinch ground nutmeg

1 cup buttermilk

1 cup blackberries (1/2 pint)

Method

1. To bloom, sprinkle gelatin with 1 Tbsp. of water. Measure the sweetener, xanthan gum, and salt in a non-reactive metal pot with a 4-6 cup size. Add the yolks and eggs and mix until thoroughly mixed. Whisk in the heavy cream and buttermilk.

2. Put the pot over medium heat until the mixture starts to thicken, whisking continuously - about 5 minutes if using Tagatesse (either a sugar) and 8 mins for Sukrin:1 or Swerve. Switch the heat medium-low and whisk for 1 minute with vigor (If whisking fails, the custard can burst). Remove from the heat and whisk for 90 seconds more. Tear the gelatin into bits and pour it into the custard and stir until it is dissolved. Include vanilla and the nutmeg, stirring until combined.

3. Only cool the mixture slowly, and pipe it onto the pre-baked pie crust. Balance the top and layer the blackberries until they are at least halfway submerged, pressing them into a custard. Refrigerate exposed before coating with cling film for several hours. Before chopping and serving, chill for at least 6 hours.

32 Low Carb Chocolate Chip Muffins

Servings: 6 | **Time**: 30 mins | **Difficulty:** Easy

Nutrients per serving: Calories: 270 kcal | Fat: 24g | Carbohydrates: 11g | Protein: 7g | Fiber: 7g

Ingredients

Cream Together:

1/2 tsp of lemon zest

1/2 tsp of vanilla extract

1/4 cup low carb sugar

2 oz softened unsalted butter

4 oz softened cream cheese

Dry Ingredients:

1 tsp baking powder

1/2 cup coconut flour

1/4 tsp salt

1/8 tsp xanthan gum

Wet Ingredients:

1/4 cup heavy cream

3 large eggs

Fold:

3 tbsp Lily's Sugar-free Chocolate Chips

4 oz strawberries, small dice

Method

1. Preheat the oven to 350 °F and place the rack in the middle. Standard muffin wells from Line 6 with paper liners. Dice some strawberries. The lemon zest. Mix the dry ingredients.

2. Cream together the whole 5 ingredients until light and smooth with a hand mixer. Again, add 1 egg and milk.

3. Apply 1/3 of the dry, well-beaten ingredients, followed by another egg. Only repeat. Make sure that a soft mousse-like appearance is preserved by fading out. The rest of the dry ingredients are added, followed by heavy cream. Half of the strawberries and half of the chocolate chips are rolled in. The batter's going to be dense.

4. Spoon the batter in a zip-lock bag and slit one of the corners with a wide hole. Squeeze the batter, placed in the middle, onto each liner. Use a muffin scoop alternately. To resist browning, brush the top of the muffins with erythritol. Arrange the remaining chocolate chips and strawberries on top.

5. In the oven center, put the muffin tin and set the oven up to 400 °F for 6 minutes. Switch the oven back to 350 °F and bake for an extra 12-18 minutes. The tops should be solid to the touch but still, look a little wet. On a wire rack, cool perfectly. Keep it softly warm in the refrigerator before eating it.

33 No-Bake Sugar-Free Strawberry Cheesecake Tart

Servings: 10 | **Time:** 35 mins | **Difficulty**: Easy

Nutrients per serving: Calories: 306 kcal | Fat: 28g | Carbohydrates: 5g | Protein: 10g | Fiber: 3g

Ingredients

Walnut Hemp Seeds Crust:

2 tbsp of coconut oil (melted)

1/2 cup Bob's Mill Hemp Seed's Hearts

1 tbsp of Sukrin Fiber Gold Syrup/Vitafiber Syrup

1 cup walnut pieces, toasted

Cheesecake Filling :

1 tbsp lemon juice

1/4 cup low carb powdered sugar

4 ounces cream cheese cold

4 ounces softened goat cheese

6 ounces strawberries, sliced zest from the lemon

4 ounces heavy cream, cold

Optional:

2 tsp fresh thyme or rosemary (finely chopped)

Method

1. The oven should be preheated to 350 °F. Put on a sheet pan and then toast the walnuts for 15 minutes or until golden in color. To remove most of the loosened skin, let it cool, then rub in the tea towel.

2. In a food processor, position the hemp seeds and the walnuts and grind them until finely ground. To spread the ingredients, apply the molten coconut oil and fiber syrup (you can use honey if not low carb), then pulse. (If rolled into balls, this also produces a perfect snack.)

3. Using parchment paper to cover a tart pan. (I used a round 14x6x1 tin, but it would fit with a big circular or many small round tins.) Spread the mixture of the crust into the pan and then force it into the crust to ensure that the sides are solid. Cover tightly and place until set in the freezer and the filling is prepared or place until appropriate in the refrigerator. It thaws rapidly.

4. In a cup, add cream cheese and the sweetener, and whip until loosened with a hand mixture. Add some heavy cream, then whip until soft and light. Finally, add the cheese from the goat and whip it again. Use or cover immediately and put in the fridge until needed. Whip to loosen before expanding onto the tart crust when kept overnight in the refrigerator. (Place 1/3 of a filling in a piping bag before piping to decorate the roof. First, we place the strawberries and decorate them around.)

5. Cut the strawberries and add the filling to them. Serve instantly. If you serve later, right before eating, apply the sliced strawberries to keep them from being soggy.

34 Black Bottom Pie

Servings: 10 | **Time**: 50 mins | **Difficulty**: Easy

Nutrients per serving: Calories: 273 kcal | Fat: 26g | Carbohydrates: 8g | Protein: 6g | Fiber: 26g

Ingredients

Base Custard:

1 recipe Low Carb Flaky Pie Crust (pre-baked)

1 tbsp gelatin

2 tsp cornstarch (or arrowroot powder)

3 large egg yolks

1 whole egg

1/2 tsp salt

1 1/4 cup heavy cream

1/4 cup water

1/4 tsp xanthan gum

2/3 cup low carb sugar

3/4 cup almond milk

Black Bottom Layer:

1 cup custard

1 1/2 oz unsweetened baking chocolate

Chiffon Layer:

remaining custard

3 large egg whites

1/2 tsp cream of tartar

1 tsp vanilla

1 tbsp rum, bourbon, or brandy

Whipped Cream Topping:

1/4 cup low carb powdered sugar

1/2 cup heavy cream

Optional:

shaved chocolate

Method

1. Separate 3 eggs into whites and yolks. Ensure the whites don't have any yolks, so they don't whip through the meringue required for the chiffon. The baking chocolate (unsweetened) is finely diced and then put in a small heat-safe bowl wide enough to hold 1 cup of custard. In a small cup, position the water and spray the gelatin over a surface to bloom.

To make the custard:

1. In a small jar, mix the 2/3 cup of sweetener, xanthan gum, cornstarch or arrowroot, and salt. Apply the egg yolks and the entire egg to the whisk. Heavy cream and almond milk are whisked in.

2. Switch the heat to low-medium. Whisk until the mixture starts to thicken, approximately 8-10 minutes, slowly but steadily, paying closer

concentration to the sides and the bottom of the pot. Whisk briskly for about 2-4 more minutes as the custard begins to cook and thicken. For an extra 2 minutes, withdraw the custard from the heating and whisk.

Black Bottom Layer:

1. Drop the hot custard from one Cup and add it to the cut chocolate. Whisk once mixed with the cocoa. Let it cool, then put it into the crust of the pie. Protect and hold refrigerated.

Chiffon Layer:

1. Tear into tiny pieces the bloomed gelatin and apply it to the leftover custard. Whisk until it melts completely with the gelatin. Coat the custard with the cling film, allowing the steam to escape from a slight gap. When it has cooled, refrigerate for 2-3 hrs.

2. Place the egg albumins in a medium bowl, then sprinkle with the tartar cream until the custard's remainder has cooled. a Whisk at medium-high speed using a hand or a stand mixer until the egg albumins quadruple in volume is shiny and maintains a stiff top when the beaters are pulled straight up from the bowl. Only put aside.

3. Take the cooled custard from the fridge and use a hand or stand mixer to whisk it to loosen its texture. Include the rum and vanilla (or the flavoring of your choice) and whip again. If you like it sweeter, now is the time to change the sugar with the powdered stevia or a stevia glycerite.

4. Apply 1/3 of the meringue to custard and use a hand mixer to combine softly. Fold half the remaining meringue with the large rubber spatula into a lightened custard. Old the leftover meringue onto the custard softly but thoroughly, finishing the chiffon layer. Now spoon into a crust of the pie and smooth out to the edges. Refrigerate for several hours until exposed. Then, cover loosely and refrigerate overnight with clinging wrap.

Whipped Cream Topping:

1. Whip the sweetener with the heavy cream until it is thick. Swirl with a whisk and spoon into the pastry. Cover it with shavings of chocolate if you like. Use a vegetable peeler to shave the cocoa, as though you're peeling a carrot.

35 Sugar-Free Carrot Cake Cupcakes

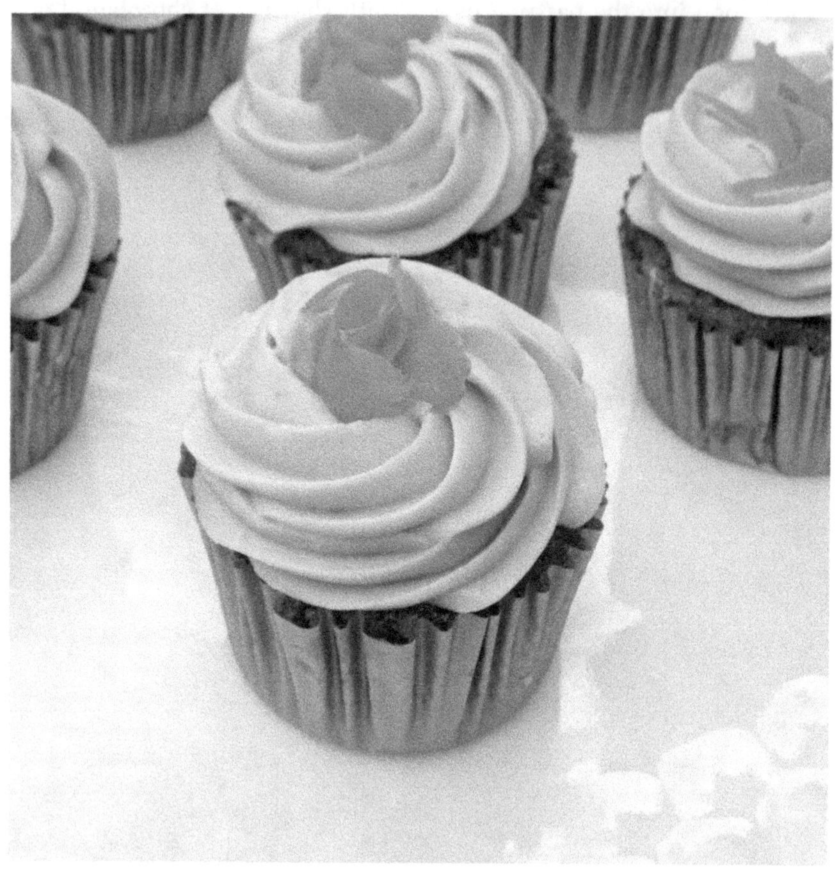

Servings: 9 | **Time:** 1 hr | **Difficulty**: Easy

Nutrients per serving: Calories: 370 kcal | Fat: 35g | Carbohydrates: 7g | Protein: 8g | Fiber: 3g

Ingredients

Cream Together:

1/3 cup Low carb brown sugar

1/2 tsp vanilla

4 tbsp butter, softened

Dry Ingredients:

1/4 cup shredded coconut

1/4 tsp ground ginger

1/4 tsp salt

1/3 cup almond flour

1/3 cup coconut flour

2 tbsp whey protein powder (helps with texture)

1 tsp baking powder

1 tsp cinnamon

Wet Ingredients:

2 ounces finely grated carrot (about 1 medium)

2 tbsp heavy cream

3 large eggs

Fluffy Cream Cheese Frosting:

1 tsp vanilla

1/2 cup heavy cream whipped very stiffly (4 oz)

1/3 cup low carb powdered sugar (or Swerve Confectioners)

4 ounces butter softened

4 ounces cream cheese softened

Method

1. Preparation: Preheat the oven to 350 °F and put the rack on the oven's bottom. Wells of Line 9 cupcakes with liners. Measure in a small bowl of dry ingredients and whisk to break up some lumps. Grate the carrot finely.

2. 2. Method: In a medium cup, place the melted butter, the brown sugar substitute, and vanilla and mix until light and fluffy with a hand mixer. Add 1 egg and beat until the mixture is light, dense, and fluffy again.

3. 3. Apply 1/3 of dry ingredients and combine properly, cleaning the Cup thoroughly. Add another egg and blend until it is mixed well and light and fluffy with the batter. After the dry additions, begin mixing the dry and wet components, rubbing the bowl and leaving the texture smooth and light. At the very top, add the carrot and the heavy cream until mixed, blend. (The batter should be moist but simple to deal with. Add 1-2 more Tsp. of heavy cream if it's not, but work quickly).

4. 4. Bake: Before it thickens, get the batter into cupcake liners. Cut the batter equally between the muffin liners, then put it in the oven. To rise the flour, turn the oven to 400 °F and bake for 5 minutes. Turn the oven back to 350 F and bake for about 20 minutes or until the tops become firm but still sound moist when gently pressed with a finger. Remove and allow to cool entirely before frosting.

5. 5. Fluffy Cream Cheese Frosting: First, whip together the vanilla extract and a sweetener with the butter and cream cheese. Until it is very stiff, whip the heavy cream. 1/3 at a time, add the whipped cream into the cream cheese mixture. Frost and refrigerate the cupcakes or serve.

36 Strawberry Cream Cheese Crumble Bars

Servings: 16 | **Time**: 45 mins | **Difficulty**: Easy

Nutrients per serving: Calories: 284 kcal | Fat: 19g | Carbohydrates: 7g | Protein: 9g | Fiber: 3g

Ingredients

Shortbread Crust:

1 1/4 tsp ground ginger

1 cup Bob's Red Mill Shredded Coconut ground

1/2 tsp salt

1/3 cup Low carb brown sugar

1/3 cup whey protein powder

2 cups almond flour

4 oz butter, melted Cream Cheese

1 large egg

1/4 cup low carb powdered sugar

8 oz cream cheese (softened)

Crumble Topping:

Low carb brown sugar optional (to taste)

8 oz strawberries (small dice)

1/3 cup sliced almonds

1 cup of reserved shortbread crust mixture

Method

1. Preheat the oven to 350°F. Spray with a baking spray on a 9 x 9-inch metal pan and line with a parchment strip that occupies all or much of the pan's bottom and overhangs the two opposite sides. After frying, this will help you extract the entire dessert from the pan. Powder the coconut in the coffee grinder. Dice some strawberries.

2. Measure into a small mixing bowl all of the dry ingredients. With a whisk, blend thoroughly. The butter is melted and added to the dry ingredients. With a broad spoon or rubber spatula, stir and press a mixture until the butter is absorbed. To verify if it can stay together nicely, pinch a small amount in your palm. If not, substitute the melted butter for 1-2 more Tsp. . Drop 1 cup of the crumble topping mixture

3. In a small cup, beat the melted cream cheese with an egg and Sukrin Melis until they are thoroughly mixed.

4. Pour the remainder of the shortbread paste into the pan, spread it thinly, and cover with a sheet of waxed paper. Use a smooth glass bottom to press the crust tightly into the pan. Low the cream cheese over the crust with a spoon and spread it carefully. Accessible areas will be there. Distribute the strawberries sliced. Over the strawberries, crumble 1/2 of a reserved crust mixture and half of the almonds. And repeat. Sprinkle with extra sweetener if needed.

5. Place in the oven center and cook for 30-40 mins or until golden brown outside. Before getting it out of the grill, let it cool down.

6. Cut a strawberry cream cheese crumble with a large chef's knife into 16 circles, chopping it straight down. Put in an airtight jar in the freezer.

37 Low Carb Raspberry Custard

Servings: 4 | **Time**: 45 mins | **Difficulty:** Easy

Nutrients per serving: Calories: 391 kcal | Fat: 34g | Carbohydrates: 6g | Protein: 5g | Fiber: 1g

Ingredients

1 2/3 cups heavy cream

1/4 tsp stevia glycerite (or more Sukrin to taste)

1/3 cup low carb powdered sugar

1/4 tsp vanilla bean powder (or 1/2 tsp vanilla extract)

1 cup Brut Champagne

6 large egg yolks

2 ounces raspberries

Method

1. Simmer over medium-low heat the champagne - low heat until only 2-3 Tbsp. are remaining. Be alert that it shouldn't burn. To cool, spill into a small glass bowl.

2. Preheat the oven to 350 °F and place the rack in the center position. Heat water until hot, but not boiling, in a tea kettle. Halfway up sides of the ramekins, find a pan wide enough to accommodate 4 ramekins and shallow enough to add water.

3. In a medium dish, apply the yolks and 1 tbsp of the sweetener. Beat well to break up the yolks entirely. Remove any residual chalazia. In a small bath, mix in the heavy cream and apply the remaining sweetener and the vanilla bean powder (add later, if using extract). Place the pot over medium heat and heat until bubbles begin to boil along the edge of the pot, stirring regularly with a whisk. Turn the heat off and start pouring the egg yolk in the hot cream mixture in a thin stream very slowly, while whisking all the while rapidly. Whisk in the champagne and stevia glycerite reduction (add the vanilla extract if you are using that instead).

4. Place each ramekin with 3 raspberries. Divide the mixture of crème Brulee equally into four ramekins. Lace the ramekins in the pan and, halfway up sides of the ramekins, fill the pan with hot water. Place the pan carefully in the oven and bake for 30 mins or until gently set at the very beginning of the crème Brulee.

5. In the water bath, cool the crème Brulee for an hour before removing it to a rack to cool fully. Cover and cool with plastic wrap for at least 4 hours (overnight is better).

6. Before eating, sprinkle 1/2 Tsp. of sweetener over the top of each crème Brulee. Use a cooking torch to heat the sweetener until it caramelizes, turning orange. Alternately, apply to the top a dollop of whipped cream. Just serve. If needed, garnish with extra raspberries. (Custards can be stored for up to 3 days in the refrigerator - no longer than that, and the raspberries start to release water).

38 Sugar-free Lemon Cupcakes with Cream Cheese Frosting

Servings: 6 | **Time:** 30 mins | **Difficulty**: Easy

Nutrients per serving: Calories: 375 kcal | Fat: 36g | Carbohydrates: 7g | Protein: 7g | Fiber: 3g

Ingredients

Whipped Cream Cheese Frosting:

4 ounces cream cheese, cold

1/4 cup low carb powdered sugar

3/4 cup heavy cream (6 oz)

Sugar-free Lemon Cupcakes

1 tbsp lemon juice

1 tsp baking powder

1/2 cup coconut flour

1/2 tsp vanilla extract

1/3 cup low carb sugar

1/4 cup heavy cream

1/4 tsp LorAnn Lemon Oil

1/4 tsp salt

2 ounces butter, soft

2 ounces cream cheese, soft

3 large eggs (cold)

zest from 1 lemon

Method

1. Cream Cheese Frosting: (The mixer works well, but a hand mixer also works.) To remove it, whip the cream cheese. Add and whip the powdered sweetener. When mixed, Mix, then whisk until the frosting is stiff and smooth by incorporating the heavy cream at a time. Use it immediately, or cover and then refrigerate until needed.

2. Preparation: The oven should be preheated to 350 °F. Place the rack in the center of the oven—the lemon with zest and juice. Line a muffin pan with 6 wells and cupcake liners. Whisk the baking powder, coconut flour, and salt together in a shallow bowl to break down any lumps. Apply the heavy cream to the lemon juice.

3. Method: Beat the first 6 ingredients of the cupcakes in a medium bowl until finely ground (1-2 minutes). Add one egg and whisk until the mixture appears light and fluffy (this can split or detach, it's okay) into the butter mixture. Apply 1/3 of the dry ingredients and blend until thoroughly combined, ensuring the soft, fluffy feel is preserved. We want to have a light and fluffy - nearly mousse-like feel throughout this process.

4. Add now another egg and mix until combined fully. Apply half the remaining dry ingredients, stirring once more. Apply the last egg, followed by one of the last dry ingredients, and beat until thoroughly integrated. Beat until the batter is moist but still soft and fluffy. Finish by adding heavy cream.

5. In a plastic zip-lock bag, spoon the dense batter and snip off an edge, making around a 3/4-1 inch opening. In a muffin liner, put the snipped corner and squeeze a batter into the fat, rounded mound, filled around 3/4 of the muffin liner. To every muffin liner, repeat, adding any batter left to those who require a little extra. On your finger, knockdown if there are any peaks. Take the pan off the counter a few inches and let it drop.

6. Bake: Place a pan in the oven. For 5 minutes, switch the oven up to 400 °F. Switch the oven back to 350 °F and bake a lemon cupcake for a further 15-20 minutes. When gently squeezed with a finger, they are ready when they feel firm, but they still sound wet. Please remove it from the oven and cool for five minutes, then gently remove it from the pan and put it on the cooling rack to cool fully before frosting.

7. Frost: Cut the tip off a zip-loc bag of a quart size and insert a wide open-star tip. Spoon the bag with the cream cheese frosting and twist the bag over the frosting. Squeeze the frosting into a spiral, starting on the cupcake's outer edge, making it narrower in diameter when piping. Scrape a frosting off and apply it back to the bag if it's not full.

8. For 5-7 days, keep the lemon cupcakes wrapped and refrigerated.

39 Low Carb Blueberry Crumble Bars

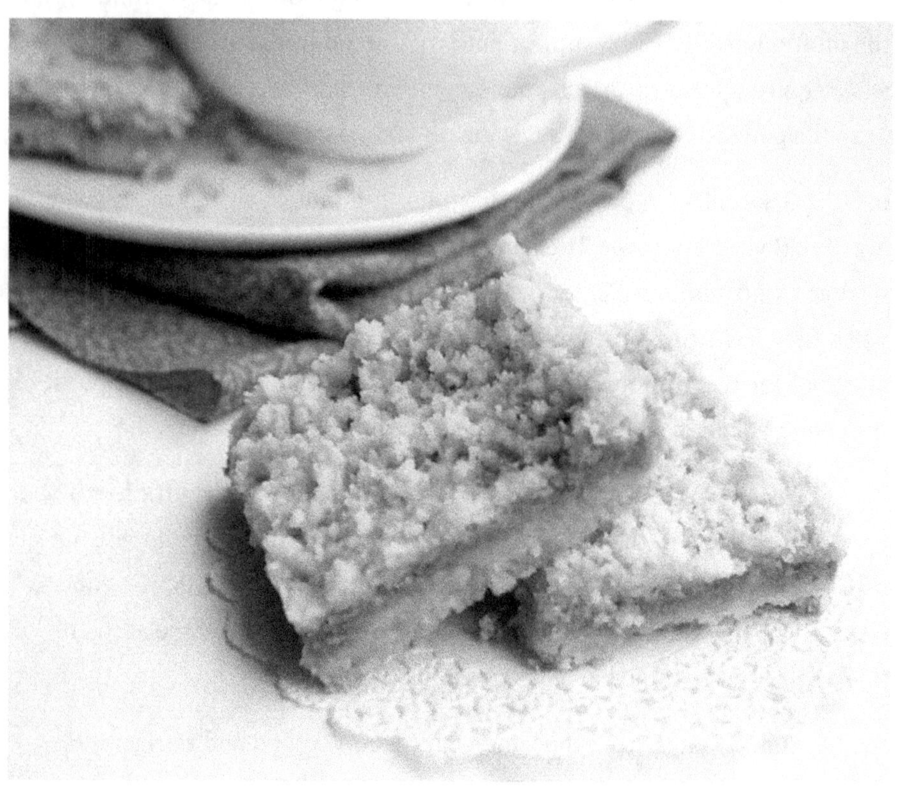

Servings: 16 | **Time:** 50 mins | **Difficulty**: Easy

Nutrients per serving: Calories: 187 kcal | Fat: 60g | Carbohydrates: 7g | Protein: 13g | Fiber: 7g

Ingredients

Shortbread Crust (reserve 1 cup for topping)

1 cup Bob's Red Mill Shredded Coconut, powdered in a coffee grinder

1/2 tsp salt

1/3 cup low carb sugar

1/3 cup whey protein powder

2 cups almond flour

9 tbsp butter, melted

Blueberry Layer:

2 cups frozen blueberries (8 oz)

1-2 pinches cinnamon

1/4 tsp xanthan gum

1/4 cup erythritol based sweetener

1 tsp cornstarch or arrowroot

1 tbsp water

1 tbsp lemon juice

Crumble Topping:

1/3 cup sliced almonds

1 cup reserved shortbread crust more sweetener to sprinkle on top

Method

1. Blueberries: In a small pot over medium heat, put the blueberries, the lemon juice, and water to thaw. Mix the egg whites. Whisk the dry ingredients into blueberries when they have been thawed and bring them to a boil, stirring until they are thickened. Leave to cool.

2. Shortbread crust: Preheat the oven to 350 ° F. Spray with a baking spray on a 9x9 inch metal pan and line with a strip of parchment that occupies all or much of the pan's bottom. And overhangs the two opposite sides, which will allow you to extract from the pan the entire dessert. Powder the coconut in the coffee grinder.

3. Measure into a small mixing bowl all the dry ingredients. With a whisk, blend thoroughly. The butter is melted and added to the dry ingredients. With a broad spoon or rubber spatula, whisk and press the mixture until the butter is integrated. To verify if it can stay together nicely, pinch a small amount in your palm. If not, substitute the melted butter for 1-2 more Tsp. .

4. Assembly: Extract the shortbread crumb solution from 1 cup. In the prepared pan, pour the mixture's remainder, scatter it thinly and cover with a sheet of waxed paper. Use a smooth glass bottom to press the crust tightly into the pan. Over the crust, pour the blueberries. Accessible areas will be there. Crumble 1/2 of the reserved crust mixture over all the blueberries and half of the almonds. And repeat. Sprinkle with extra sweetener if needed.

5. Bake: Put in the oven center and cook for about 30-40 minutes or until golden brown outside. Before getting it out of the grill, let it cool down.

6. Cut the blueberry crumble with a wide chef's knife into 16 circles, breaking it down straight. Store in an airtight jar in the freezer.

40 Low Carb Chocolate Truffle

Servings: 4 | **Time**: 40 mins | **Difficulty**: Easy

Nutrients per serving: Calories: 605 kcal | Fat: 60g | Carbohydrates: 10g | Fiber: 2g

Ingredients

Low Carb Chocolate Truffle Creme Brulee:

Ghirardelli Midnight Reserve Chocolate bar 90% or 86%

5 large egg yolks

2 tbsp good Brandy

2 cups heavy cream (16 oz)

1/3 cup low carb sugar divided

1/2 tsp stevia glycerite

Optional Toppings:

whipped cream

additional sweetener for sprinkling on top

Method

1. Preparation: Preheat the oven to 350 °F and put the rack in the center. Heat water until hot, not boiling, in a tea kettle. To suit the 4, 6-ounce ramekins, find a pan wide enough and shallow enough to add water halfway up the ramekins' sides. Get chocolate sliced into slivers.

2. Method: In a medium dish, add the yolks and 1 Tbsp. of the granulated sweetener. Beat well to break up the yolks entirely.

3. In a small pot, mix in the heavy cream and apply the leftover granulated sweetener and stevia glycerite. Put the pot over medium heat and heat until bubbles begin to boil along the edge of the pot, stirring regularly with a whisk. Turn the heat off and start pouring the egg yolk into a hot cream mixture - in a thin stream very slowly, while whisking all the while rapidly. To melt and mix, add the sliced chocolate and stir. Whisk the brandy up.

4. Bake: Split equally amongst 4 ramekins with the chocolate truffle cream Brulee mixture. Place the ramekins in the pan and, halfway up sides of the ramekins, fill the pan with hot water. Place the pan carefully in the oven and bake for about 30 minutes or until the creme brulee is lightly jiggly at the middle.

5. In the water bath, cool a chocolate truffle creme brulee for an hour before transferring it to a rack to cool completely. Cover and refrigerate for at least 4 hours with plastic wrap, but it's safer overnight.

6. Sprinkle over the top of each cream Brulee with 1/2 Tsp. Lakanto Monkfruit Sweetener or a Swerve Granulated until serving. Use a cooking torch to heat the sweetener until it caramelizes, turning orange. Alternately, apply to the top a dollop of whipped cream. Now serve.

41 Sugar-Free Coffee Creme Brulee

Servings: 4 | **Time:** 35 mins | **Difficulty**: Easy

Nutrients per serving: Calories: 510 kcal | Fat: 51g | Carbohydrates: 4.5g | Protein: 7g

Ingredients

6 large egg yolks

2 cups heavy whipping cream

1/4 tsp stevia glycerite

1/4 cup low carb sugar divided

1 tbsp V.S.O.P Brandy (or rum)

1 tbsp plus 1 tsp instant espresso

Optional Toppings:

whipped cream cinnamon

additional sweetener for melting on top

Method

1. Preparation: Preheat the oven to 350 °F and put the rack in the center. Heat water until hot, not boiling, in a tea kettle. Find a pan wide enough to accommodate the 4 ramekins, and halfway up sides of the ramekins, deep enough to add water.

2. Method: In a medium dish, add the yolks and 1 Tbsp. of the granulated sweetener. Beat well to break up the yolks entirely.

3. In a small cup, pour the heavy cream and add the left granulated sweetener, stevia glycerite, and espresso. Place the pot over medium heat and heat until bubbles begin to boil along the edge of the pot, stirring regularly with a whisk. Turn the heat off and keep pouring the egg yolk into a hot cream mixture - in a thin stream very slowly, while whisking all the while rapidly. Whisk the brandy up.

4. Bake: Divide equally amongst 4 ramekins with the coffee cream brulee mixture. Place the ramekins in the pan and, halfway up sides of the ramekins, fill the pan with hot water. Place the pan carefully in the oven and then bake for about 30 minutes or until the creme brulee is slightly jiggly at the very middle - about the size of a nickel or a dime.

5. In the water bath, cool the sugar-free coffee creme brulee for an hour before shifting it to a rack to cool fully. Cover and refrigerate for at least 4 hours with plastic wrap, but it's safer overnight.

6. Sprinkle over the top of each cream Brulee with 1/2 Tsp. Lakanto Monkfruit Sweetener or a Swerve Granulated until serving. Use a cooking torch to heat the sweetener until it caramelizes, turning orange. Instead, apply a dollop of whipped cream and some cinnamon to the tip. Now serve.

42 Low Carb Chocolate Cheesecake With Peanut Butter Mousse

Servings: 8 | **Time:** 6 hrs | **Difficulty:** Easy

Nutrients per serving: Calories: 499 kcal | Fat: 47g | Carbohydrates: 9g | Protein: 11g | Fiber: 5g

Ingredients

3 ounces Lily's Original Dark Chocolate (finely chopped)

2 Tbsp. Cocoa powder

2 Eggs

16 ounces Cream Cheese, softened

1 cup Swerve Confectioners Sugar Substitute

1 cup Keto Peanut Butter Mousse

⅔ Cup Sour cream

½ Tbsp. Vanilla

Method

1. Preheat the oven to 350°F.
2. By oiling it with butter or a non-stick spray and lined the bottom with the piece of parchment paper, prepare a 6-inch springform sheet. Use aluminum foil to seal the exterior of the springform pan and place it in an

oven bag. This bag should not cover the pan's surface, but you can fold it down based on its height so that it only meets the top lip of a springform pan.

3. Place the mixer bowl with the melted cream cheese and blend until smooth and fluffy. Apply the combination of sour cream and vanilla until well mixed.

4. Whisk the powdered sugar alternative and cocoa powder together in a shallow cup. Add with cream cheese mixture and blend until thoroughly mixed.

5. In a microwave-safe cup, put Lily's dark chocolate and microwave for 10 secs, stirring in it each time until melted and smooth. Let the cream cheese mixture cool for 1 min and then pour it in, stirring until it is completely mixed.

6. Add the eggs one at a time and blend until each egg is mixed. Only don't overmix. In the 6-inch springform bath, pour the mixture into it.

7. Bake it in a bath of water. In a wider bath, sit the springform pan (a roasting pan, deep casserole dish, or a disposable foil pan is best). Flush the pan with water before the side of a springform pan hits 1 -1.5 inches upwards.

8. Place in the oven, then bake for 45-60 minutes or until just barely jiggly in the very middle. Turn the oven off and open the door to allow the cheesecake to cool for 30 minutes. Remove it from the oven and let it cool at room temperature perfectly.

9. Remove it from a springform and wrap the parchment paper collar across it when the cheesecake is cooled. The sheet of parchment paper long and approximately two inches longer than the cake to fit around the edge of the cake. Tape together the ends such that the parchment paper remains in place.

10. Create the mousse with keto peanut butter and spread it over the cheesecake's top. It would be stopped from running off the side by the parchment paper.

11. Put in the fridge for a minimum of 4 hours to cool, preferably overnight. Until eating, take the parchment paper and enjoy it.

43 Low Carb Blackberry Pudding

Servings: 2 | **Time:** 5 mins | **Difficulty**: Easy

Nutrients per serving: Calories: 459.5 kcal | Fat: 44.04g | Carbohydrates: 4.91g | Protein: 9.1g | Fiber: 5.75 g

Ingredients

1/4 cup Coconut Flour

1/4 tsp. Baking Powder

1/4 cup Blackberries

5 large Egg Yolks

2 tbsp. Coconut Oil

2 tbsp. Butter

2 tbsp. Heavy Cream

2 tsp. Lemon Juice Zest

1 Lemon

2 tbsp. Erythritol

10 drops Liquid Stevia

Method

1. Preheat the oven to 350 °F.

2. Separate the egg yolks from the egg whites and set aside the yolks. Measure out and set aside the dry ingredients. Measure and set aside the butter and the coconut oil.

3. Beat the egg yolks until the color is pale, then add the erythritol and stevia. Beat once more before well mixed.

4. Add lemon juice, heavy cream, lemon zest, butter, and coconut oil. Beat again before completely mixed.

5. Sift dry ingredients over ingredients that are damp and blend well again.

6. Between 2 ramekins, spread the batter, then press 2 tbsp—blackberries in any single ramekin. Before moving them into the batter, you want to gently smash the blackberries with the finger.

7. Bake, let cool for 20-25 minutes, and then enjoy

44 Low Carb Chocolate Peanut Butter Cookies

Servings: 10 | **Time:** 25 mins | **Difficulty**: Easy

Nutrients per serving: Calories: 230 kcal | Fat: 20g | Carbohydrates: 6g | Protein: 6g | Fiber: 2g

Ingredients

1 tsp Vanilla Extract

1 Egg, large

2 tbsps Cocoa Powder, unsweetened

10 Sugar-free Peanut Butter Cups

1 1/2 c Bob's Red Mill Fine Almond Flour

1/4 c Unsalted Butter, softened

1/4 c Sucralose granulated sweetener

1/4 tsp Baking Soda

1/4 tsp Salt

Method

1. Combine the cocoa powder, almond flour, baking soda, and salt in a shallow cup. Only put aside.

2. Cream the butter and sweetener in a blender until smooth, around 2 minutes.

3. Stir in the butter with the egg and vanilla and proceed to blend.

4. Gently add dry ingredients to a bowl before all the ingredients are thoroughly combined, then begin to blend.

5. Preheat the oven to 350 °F.

6. Scoop 2 tbsp of dough from the bowl and shape a sugar-free cup of peanut butter around it. If all of the dough is used, repeat this process.

7. Put on a lined baking sheet with cookies and then bake for bout 10-12 minutes.

8. Let the cookies on the baking sheet chill for 5 minutes, then switch them to a cooling rack for cooling completely.

45 Spicy Chocolate Cookie Truffles

Servings: 2 | **Time:** 1 hr 35 mins | **Difficulty**: Easy

Nutrients per serving: Calories: 152 kcal | Fat: 14g | Carbohydrates: 4g | Protein: 2g | Fiber: 2g

Ingredients

Toothpicks optional

4 oz. cream cheese softened

3 Tbsp. cocoa

1/3 cup Monkfruit blend sweetener

1 tsp. vanilla

1 Tbsp. coconut flour

1 oz. cream cheese softened

1 cup almond flour

1 1/2 tsp. coconut oil

1 ½ cups sugar-free semi-sweet baking chips

½ cup salted butter softened

¼ tsp. Salt

¼ tsp. cayenne pepper

Method

1. Whisk in the butter and 1 ounce Of cream cheese for each other. Add and beat the sweetener before well added. Mix the vanilla in it. Apply the salt, chocolate, coconut flour, and pepper to the almond flour and blend until well mixed. On a parchment sheet or plastic wrap, put the dough and shape into a log about 2-1/2 inches in diameter. In the freezer, seal, and ice, or freeze until solid.

2. Cut the dough into 1/4 inch slices and put on a baking sheet lined with parchment. Bake for 15-20 minutes at 325. If you take them out of the oven, the cookies will be tender but will tighten up as they cool on the plate. Leave the cookies on the sheet pan to cool perfectly.

3. Add the cookies to the bowl of the food processor and pulse until crumbs are formed. Add four ounces Of cream cheese, then pulse until it forms a dough. Divide the dough into 20 mounds using a cookie scoop and put it on the parchment-lined pan you have used for your cookies. To smooth it out, roll each ball in your palm. For about twenty minutes or until stable, freeze the dough balls.

4. Merge the baking chips and the coconut oil in a mug or small bowl and microwave at intervals of 15 seconds until melted and smooth. At the top of each ball, put a toothpick (use as a stick). Dip into the melting chocolate for coating. And let excess drip off and put it back on the pan lined with parchment. For both of the balls, repeat. Until set, refrigerate. When the chocolate shell dries, carefully rotate the toothpick to clear any residual molten chocolate and drizzle with it.

46 Keto Rice Pudding

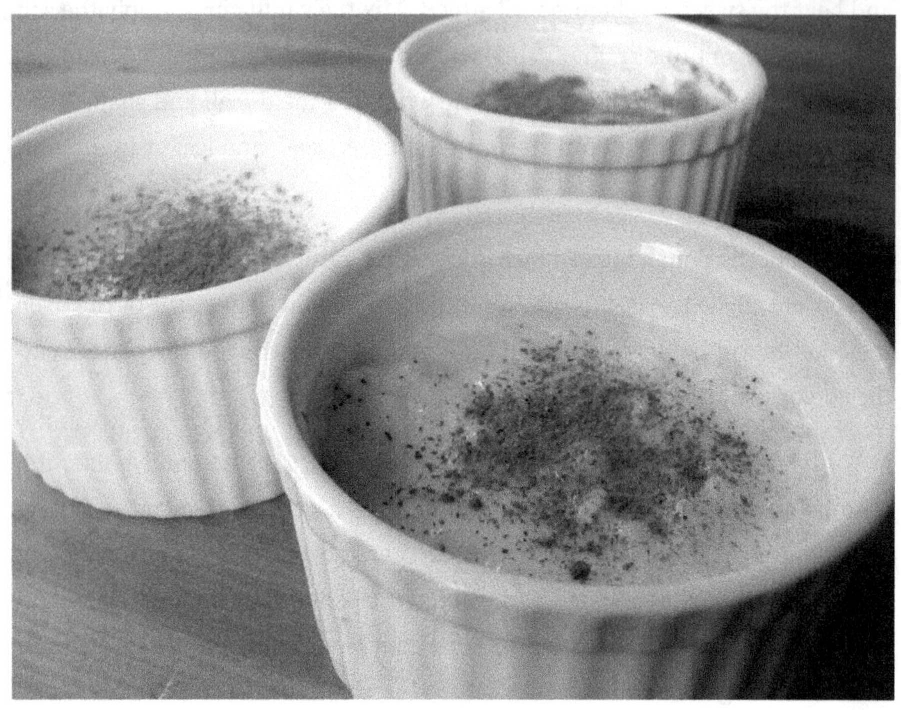

Servings: 4 | **Time:** 4 hrs 15 mins | **Difficulty**: Easy

Nutrients per serving: Calories: 228 kcal | Fat: 20g | Carbohydrates: 6g | Protein: 4g | Fiber: 1g

Ingredients

Pinch salt

1 cup cauliflower rice, steamed (cooled and pressed dry)

4 large egg yolks, beaten

1 tsp. vanilla

1/2 cup unsweetened almond milk

1/2 tsp. ground cinnamon

1/3 cup Allulose Blend Sweetener

1/4 tsp. cardamom

1 can (13.5 oz) full fat coconut milk

Method

1. Combine the coconut milk, almond milk, sweetener, cardamom, salt, cinnamon, cauliflower rice, and egg yolks in a medium saucepan. Heat the mixture softly, stirring continuously over medium- low pressure. For 7-10 minutes, continue cooking, stirring continuously, until the mixture dense and reaches 170-180°F. Don't let it simmer in the mixture. The back of a spoon should coat the mixture.

2. Withdraw from the sun. Add the vanilla and pour it into four serving bowls. Cover and chill until set, around 4 hours, with plastic wrap—store for up to 3 days in the fridge.

47 Keto Cranberry Brie Tart

Servings: 20 | **Time:** 27 mins | **Difficulty**: Easy

Nutrients per serving: Calories: 171 kcal | Fat: 14g | Carbohydrates: 5g | Protein: 7g | Fiber: 2g

Ingredients

1 cup coconut flour

2 Tbsp. Monfruit/ Erythritol Blend Sweetener

Zest from one small navel orange

2 oz. cream cheese

2 eggs

18 oz. double cream brie cheese rind removed

1/8 Tsp. cayenne

1/4 Tsp. paprika

1/4 cup toasted chopped pecans

1 jalapeno finely diced

1 ½ Tsp. apple cider vinegar

1 ½ cup fresh cranberries

½ Tsp. salt

½ cup of water

½ cup Monkfruit/Erythritol Blend Sweetener

½ cup butter cold and cut into pieces

¼ Tsp. paprika

Method

1. Combine the coconut flour, sweetener, spices, and salt in a food processor and pulse to combine. Apply the eggs, cream cheese, and slices of cold butter and pulse until the mixture gets together and away from the bowl's edges. Place them in a plastic wrap and cool for 30 minutes.

2. Press the dough uniformly into a tart pan that has been gently sprayed. Bake for 20 minutes at 325 °F or until it is golden. Set to cool aside.

3. In a saucepan, mix the cranberries, jalapeno, water, vinegar, sweetener, orange zest, and paprika and bring a boil over medium heat to simmer. Simmer for almost 5 minutes or before the mixture thickens, and the cranberries erupt. Remove the orange zest and chill for at least 30 minutes in the refrigerator before it cools.

4. Place the brie into a bowl of a stand mixer, with the rinds cut. Beat around 5-7 minutes or until it becomes smooth and silky with a paddle attachment at low velocity. Scrape down the sides as appropriate, every minute. Only put aside.

5. Spread uniformly over the bottom of a crust with the whipped brie. Next, the cranberry sauce is poured over the top of the brie. Sprinkle and serve with toasted pecans, then slice. Store in the fridge while covered.

48 Keto Molasses Cookies

Servings: 24 | **Time:** 18 mins | **Difficulty**: Easy

Nutrients per serving: Calories: 89 kcal | Fat: 8g | Carbohydrates: 3g | Protein: 2g | Fiber: 2g

Ingredients

2 Tbsp. coffee flour

1/8 tsp. black pepper

1/3 cup + 2 Tbsp. Monkfruit/Erythritol Blend Sweetener like Lakanto

1 Tsp. cinnamon

1 Tbsp. grass-fed gelatin powder

1 egg

1 ½ Tsp. ground ginger

1 ¼ cup almond flour

¾ Tsp. baking soda

½ Tsp. vanilla extract

½ Tsp. ground clove

½ cup butter

¼ Tsp. salt

¼ cup of creamy almond butter (well stirred & room temperature)

Method

1. Preheat the oven to 375°F.

2. Combine the sugar, sweetener, and almond butter and beat until well mixed. In the egg, mix. Mix well with the almond flour, baking soda, salt, coffee flour, gelatin, ginger clove, cinnamon, vanilla, and pepper. For 15-20 minutes, refrigerate the dough.

3. Scoop the dough onto a sheet pan lined with parchment and bake for about 8 minutes. Cool in the jar. Store the cookies at room temperature in a sealed jar.

49 Keto Lemon Loaf Cake

Servings: 12 | **Time:** 55 mins | **Difficulty:** Easy

Nutrients per serving: Calories: 173 kcal | Fat: 16g | Carbohydrates: 4g | Protein: 6g | Fiber: 2g

Ingredients

Zest of 2 lemons

4 oz cream cheese softened

4 eggs room temperature

2 Tsp. baking powder

2 Tbsp. coconut flour

1/4 cup butter softened

1/2 Tsp. salt

1/2 cup Lakanto Monkfruit Sweetener or equivalent sweetener of choice

1 Tsp. vanilla extract

1 1/2 cup almond flour

Method

1. Preheat a 350 °F oven and oil a 9-5-inch loaf pan. Only put aside,

2. Combine the almond flour, baking powder, coconut flour, and salt in a medium dish.

3. Cream butter with a sweetener in the large mixing bowl until smooth & fluffy. Add the cream cheese and blend to ensure no lumps.

4. Add the eggs one at a time to the butter mixture, combining thoroughly after each addition. Include vanilla and zest.

5. For butter and eggs, add the dry ingredients to the mixture. Mix well before blended well.

6. Load the batter into a 9-5 inch oiled loaf bowl. For 40-45 minutes, bake. After 30 minutes, start testing for density.

7. Remove from the oven and leave to cool for 25 minutes, then cool fully on the rack before slicing.

50 Keto Chocolate Zucchini Bread

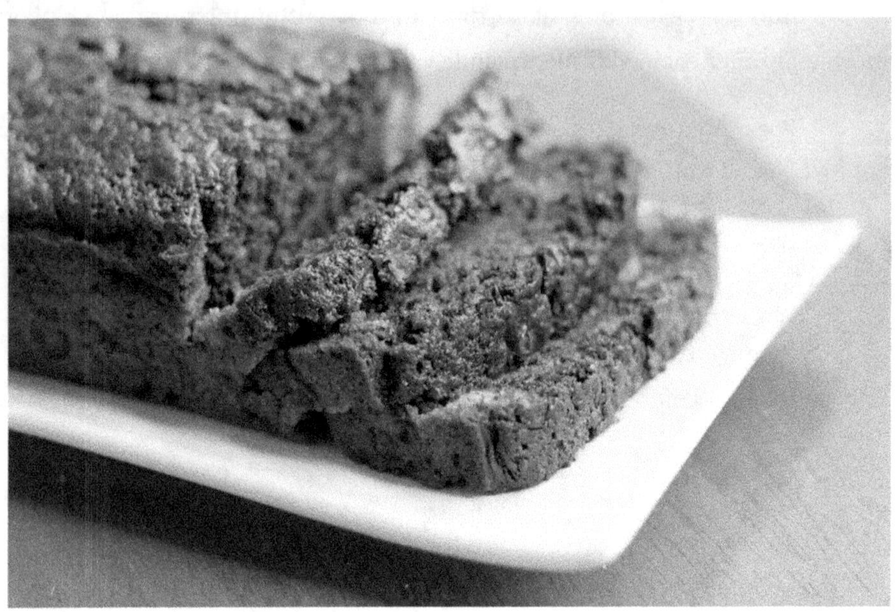

Servings: 16 | **Time:** 55 mins | **Difficulty:** Easy

Nutrients per serving: Calories: 153 kcal | Fat: 13g | Carbohydrates: 8g | Protein: 6g | Fiber: 4g

Ingredients

1 cup almond flour

1 cup grated zucchini

1 tsp. baking soda

1 tsp. vanilla extract

1/2 cup coconut flour

1/2 cup sugar-free semi-sweet chocolate chips (divided)

1/2 tsp salt

1/4 cup + 2 Tbsp. cocoa

11/2 tsp. baking powder

3/4 cup Lakanto Golden Monkfruit Sweetener

6 Tbsp. butter, ghee or coconut oil, melted

8 eggs

Method

1. Preheat the oven to 350°C. Oiled and 8-9″ loaf pan with parchment or spray.

2. Combine the coconut flour and almond flour, and the other 5 ingredients in a small bowl and whisk well to blend. Only put aside.

3. Whip eggs until light & foamy triples in volume using the stand mixer and then whisk. This can also be accomplished with a handheld mixer, but to reduce splatter, use a big bowl.

4. Turn to the paddle attachment if a stand mixer is used. Add the eggs to the mixture of almond flour and blend properly. To the egg mixture, apply the rubbed zucchini, extract and the melted butter and whisk at a medium pace until mixed, scratching the sides at least once. Stir in the reserved chocolate chips with 1 Tbsp. Up to the end of the loaf.

5. Now spoon the batter into a prepared loaf pan uniformly and smooth the top out. Sprinkle with the remainder of 1 Tbsp. Chips uniformly around the batter's top. Bake for 45 minutes to one hour at 350°F or until a tester looks clean. "The baking time is slightly shorter if you use a 9" plate, so keep an eye on it, starting for 30 minutes

6. Cool in the skillet. Take the loaf out from the pan and slice with the parchment. Enjoy a cup of coffee. This bread can be rolled and placed in the refrigerator or frozen completely or in slices.

www.ingramcontent.com/pod-product-compliance
Lightning Source LLC
Chambersburg PA
CBHW071446030726
47593CB00003B/914

* 9 7 8 1 8 0 2 7 7 1 7 2 5 *